Instructor's Manual for
Ignatavicius & Workman

Medical-Surgical Nursing: Critical Thinking for Collaborative Care

4th edition

Susan Nickell Behmke, MS, RN
Professor of Nursing and Level I Coordinator
College of Southern Maryland
La Plata, Maryland

Sharon Souter, MSN, RN
Director of Nursing
New Mexico State University at Carlsbad
Carlsbad, New Mexico

Donna D. Ignatavicius, MS, RN, Cm
President, DI Associates, Inc.
Hughesville, Maryland
Former Professor
Charles County Community College
La Plata, Maryland

W.B. Saunders Company

Philadelphia London Montreal Sydney Tokyo Toronto

W.B. Saunders Company

The Curtis Center
Independence Square West
Philadelphia, Pennsylvania 19106-3399

Vice President and Publishing Director, Nursing: Sally Schrefer
Executive Editor: Robin Carter
Managing Editor: Lee Henderson
Project Manager: Gayle Morris
Production Editor: Stephanie M. Hebenstreit
Designer: Teresa Breckwoldt

Instructor's Manual for Medical-Surgical Nursing: Critical Thinking for Collaborative Care, FOURTH EDITION

International Standard Book Number: 0-7216-8764-4

NOTICE

Medical-surgical nursing is an ever-changing field. Standard safety precautions must be followed, but as new research and clinical experience broaden our knowledge, changes in treatment and drug therapy may become necessary or appropriate. Readers are advised to check the most current product information provided by the manufacturer of each drug to be administered to verify the recommended dose, the method and duration of administration, and the contraindications. It is the responsibility of the appropriately licensed health care provider, relying on experience and knowledge of the patient, to determine dosages and the best treatment for each individual patient. Neither the Publisher nor the editor assume any liability for any injury and/or damage to persons or property arising from this publication.

Printed in the United States of America

01 02 03 04 05 FG/EB 9 8 7 6 5 4 3 2 1

INTRODUCTION

PHILOSOPHY AND FRAMEWORK FOR THE *INSTRUCTOR'S MANUAL*

The authors have found that most instructor's manuals are not particularly helpful. The bulk of these manuals are content outlines that reiterate the topical headings of the accompanying textbook, rather than tools that assist faculty with ideas for teaching/learning activities or resources. Therefore, the authors of this instructor's manual have designed a practical, more useful tool that will help both new and seasoned faculty focus on learning rather than teaching. This tool fosters critical thinking in students rather than merely supplementing faculty lectures.

Teaching Versus Learning

Faculty in higher education institutions spend most of their time engaging in teaching activities. The assumption is that teaching will result in learning (Anderson, 1996). However, students can learn without being taught; conversely, they sometimes do not learn even if they are taught.

Higher education has stressed the importance of teaching, yet students need to know how to learn and to make a commitment to lifelong learning. A major paradigm shift is underway as colleges and universities begin to focus more on learning and learning outcomes.

In a teaching institution, the faculty provide instruction and strive to improve the quality of the instruction. In a learning institution, faculty produce learning and strive to improve the the quality of learning. In a teaching institution, learning is teacher-centered and controlled, competitive, and individualistic. In a learning institution, learning is student-centered and controlled, cooperative, collaborative, and supportive. Faculty are primarily lecturers when teaching is emphasized; faculty are designers of learning methods and environments when learning is emphasized (Barr & Tagg, 1995).

Students and Faculty Behaviors Regarding Teaching and Learning

In the author's experience, students and faculty typically view teaching and learning from very different perspectives. Differences in developmental approaches to learning and other factors most likely explain these varying views.

For example, students complain about lack of time for learning due to family and work role obligations. Many only want to know what is expected to pass written examinations and to do well in the clinical laboratory. Prior experiences and learning opportunities also influence how students view teaching and learning. In pre-nursing courses, each educational experience is separate from others. Few courses, if any, are applied in any way to professional nursing practice. Course objectives typically measure cognitive learning. Consequently, most students enter the clinical nursing courses at a concrete thinking level. They have failed to make a connection between scientific concepts and how to apply them in a clinical situation.

Faculty members expect students to be able to function at a formal operations level, a higher level of thinking and learning. In nursing education, affective and psychomotor learning become as important as cognitive learning. Faculty may be reluctant to try new or unique activities that help students reach this next level. It is often easier for instructors to lecture to students or use other traditional teaching methods. Students are provided with a course syllabus, which includes page numbers for readings from their textbooks. This type of "feeding" behavior by faculty does not promote critical thinking in students.

New methods of teaching/learning sometimes result in poor student evaluations of faculty performance. In a system that rewards faculty based primarily on student course evaluations, faculty may not take the risks of seeking new ideas or avoiding "feeding" the students.

Critical Thinking to Promote Learning

Critical thinking has been stressed in schools of nursing for the past decade or more. As a result of the Delphi research project sponsored by the American Philosophical Association (APA) (1990), a consensus definition of critical thinking was formulated. In general, critical thinking can be characterized as purposeful, self-regulatory judgment. As a human cognitive process, critical thinking may be evident in problem solving, decision making, and clinical reasoning as part of professional practice (Facione & Facione, 1996). Mastery of critical thinking is evident when students "connect the dots," "put the puzzle pieces together," or simply experience the "ah-ha" phenomenon.

Various levels of critical thinking can be achieved. At the basic level, the learner is able to distinguish right from wrong by relying on established rules or norms. The higher-level thinker recognizes that several alternatives exist, but does not select any of these choices. The highest-level thinker, the complex critical thinker, recognizes the alternatives and selects one or more depending on the specific nature of the situation. Faculty are instrumental in helping their students develop critical thinking skills.

Many articles and books have discussed the characteristics of critical thinkers, with accompanying discussions about whether critical thinking skills can be learned or enhanced. The authors believe that critical thinking skills can be mastered and offer numerous strategies throughout this manual to help faculty foster critical thinking.

The critical thinking skills proposed by the 1990 APA Consensus Definition serve as a framework for the learning outcomes used in this manual. Table 1-1 lists these skills and sub-skills.

An emphasis on learning promotes critical thinking. The Learning Plans that accompany each unit of *Medical-Surgical Nursing: Critical Thinking for Collaborative Care,* 4th edition, provide faculty with critical thinking tools and strategies that promote learning. A comprehensive bibliography (annotated) at the end of this Introduction includes numerous articles and books that serve as additional resources for critical thinking.

COMPONENTS OF THE *INSTRUCTOR'S MANUAL*

Learning Outcomes

Each unit contains several chapters. Critical learning outcomes are provided for each unit. The learning objectives in this manual are identical to those at the beginning of each chapter in the text. Each unit also includes suggested learning activities to assist learners to accomplish the learning objectives, and a list of supplemental resources. Each unit chapter is arranged in a three-column format.

TABLE 1-1. Consensus List of Critical Thinking Cognitive Skills and Sub-Skills*

Skill	Sub-Skills
1. Interpretation	• Categorization • Decoding Significance • Clarifying Meaning
2. Analysis	• Examining Ideas • Identifying Arguments • Analyzing Arguments
3. Evaluation	• Assessing Claims • Assessing Arguments
4. Inference	• Querying Evidence • Conjecturing Alternatives • Drawing Conclusions
5. Explanation	• Stating Results • Justifying Procedures • Presenting Arguments
6. Self-regulation	• Self-examination • Self-correction

*Facione, P., project director. Critical thinking: A statement of expert consensus for purposes of educational assessment and instruction. The Delphi report: Research findings and recommendations prepared for the American Philosophical Association (ERIC Doc. No. ED315-423). Washington: *ERIC,* 1990, 12.

Learning Activities

For each critical learning outcome, there are learning activities to accomplish the outcome. The learning activities are specifically designed to help the learner acquire critical thinking skills as well as nursing knowledge. The instructor's manual identifies learning strategies that encourage learner participation such as cooperative learning structures, group activities, concept and correlation maps, algorithms, learner workbook activities, and other tips for structuring learning experience.

Learning strategies that involve group work have directions for setting up, monitoring, and closing the exercises. The authors recommend time frames for any group exercise to assist instructors in planning their time. In addition, learning strategies that are particularly suitable for distance learning are identified.

Supplemental Resources

The instructor's manual provides instructors with supplemental instructional resources such as selected transparency masters, Internet resources, materials from community organizations, and similar material. The supplementary material is recommended for independent learner exploration and learning.

STRATEGIES

Cooperative Learning Structures

Cooperative learning has been defined as "a set of instructional strategies, which include cooperative student-student interaction over subject matter as *an integral part of the learning process.*" (Kagan, 1989, p. 4:1). Cooperative learning requires that attention be focused on both the cognitive and the affective aspects of the learning experience. Team building is as important an activity as any knowledge drill, especially in the nursing profession. Learners are expected to interact with others and to promote positive relations in the learning environment. There are a vast number of cooperative learning exercises in the literature, with more being published every year. Some exercises may take as little time as 3 to 5 minutes, whereas others may span several class or clinical periods.

Group Activities

Helping learners to examine their thinking helps them with problem solving and thus with critical thinking. Frequently, learners do not know "what they don't know" until they are confronted by a different interpretation or point of view. Games, constructive controversy, quick checks such as Think-Pair-Share, and other active learner-to-learner encounters increase the opportunities that learners have to find what they know and what they don't know. Further, learners have more opportunities to make links between current and previous learning and life experiences. An old education axiom "He [or she] who explains, learns" provides a powerful rationale for instructors to listen and for learners to construct knowledge.

A second and equally compelling reason for using structured group activities is that learning to work effectively in groups with people of differing backgrounds and abilities is essential to success in nursing. Being held accountable only for one's own work is poor preparation for collaborative health team interactions. Health care, particularly nursing, demands that practitioners be able to effectively delegate tasks and supervise the work of other members of the health team. Learning social skills such as being able to disagree agreeably takes both opportunity and practice. Structured group work provides the opportunity to perfect social skills that improve group effectiveness.

Group interaction can take place in small classrooms, large lecture halls, on site, or at remote sites via distance-learning technologies. Imaginative problem solving and use of cooperative learning helps instructors structure group activities regardless of the physical environment.

Graphic Organizers

Graphic organizers such as concept maps (attribute wheels), correlation maps (webs), and algorithms (sequence chains) provide a visual window into the learner's conceptualization of knowledge. Such visual representations assist learners with "seeing" the connections between isolated pieces of information. They can also help faculty understand where the learner has difficulty. It has been the authors' experience that learners frequently complete required assignments as a series of tasks to be completed. They fail to perceive the project as a puzzle with pieces to be found to complete a larger "total" picture.

Algorithms are particularly useful for assessment tasks by helping learners to visualize if-then relationships. Concept maps are useful for assisting learners to look at all the component pieces of concepts. Clinical correlation maps assist learners to "tie all the pieces together."

Journals

Research supports the belief that directed writing facilitates learner reflection. The act of capturing thought on paper forces the writer to make conscious decisions, and to think about thinking. Journals have historically been used to examine thinking. Much of our understanding of history, for example, has come from the analysis of personal journals. Journals may be reflected upon in private or publicly in groups.

Journaling assignments may include tasks such as writing a summary or a critique, or presenting a focused argument by taking a position for or against an issue. Depending on the type of journaling assignment, learners will have practice with different critical thinking skills such as interpreting, analyzing, or explaining.

SUPPLEMENTAL RESOURCES

Transparency Masters

The transparency masters are instructional supplements for selected learning activities and are designed for whole-group instruction. The transparencies are not duplicated in other instructor resources.

Internet Resources

Internet resources are both learner- and instructor-oriented. Some Internet addresses, such as webTeacher.org, provide instructors from all disciplines with excellent advice and links for using Internet assignments with learners. Other sources provide pertinent information on a variety of topics such as search engines and criteria for evaluating Internet information resources. Other valuable information can be obtained from list servers that link educators seeking peer information ("How do you . . . in your program?"). Internet addresses are identified with suggested learner objectives and exercises. The authors strongly recommend that instructors "try out" the Internet learning activities and addresses to become familiar with them prior to making student assignments. In many instances, learners will be the instructor's best resource for Internet "how-to" advice.

Electronic mail or "e-mail" is an effective tool for instructor-learner communication. Incorporating asynchronous dialog into other learner-learner or instructor-learner communication methods helps to personalize the learning environment. E-mail among colleagues serves to help them keep abreast of current issues and to quickly find resources. One list server specifically for nurse educators is www.cod.edu/dept/Software/Favorite.htm. Subscription to list servers will bring mail every day. Many of the topics may not be of interest, but will provide a quick window into the concerns of nurse educators both nationally and internationally.

Community Organizations and Resources

Community organizations have a wealth of free material to facilitate learning. Learners need to know what is available and where to find materials for themselves and their clients. Many national organizations have Internet sites and material that can be downloaded and used immediately.

GENERAL GUIDELINES

The authors have used all of the strategies that follow. There is no presumption that the strategies are the only ones available, or even that any one is good in all circumstances. Our goal is to provide enough detail in these instructions that both novice and seasoned instructors will find some new strategies to assist learners with the hard work of learning and thinking.

Cooperative Learning Structures

Learners may need to move around in order to get into groups; clear direction is mandatory. Learners need to know where to go, who should go, and what should be done upon arrival. Time is required for movement and for settling in. Consequently, structures that require learners to move should be used judiciously.

Structures

Think-Pair-Share (Good for distance learning)
- Instructor poses question
- Learners think out their answer (approx. 1 minute)
- Two learners share their answers (2 minutes)
- One of the pair shares answer with the large group

Pairs Check (Good for distance learning)
- Learner 1 practices skills (classroom or skills laboratory)
- Learner 2 monitors and coaches
- Learner 1 and 2 reverse roles
- After each learner has practiced, pairs check with another pair

Numbered Heads Together (Good for distance learning)
- Learners count off by fours
- Instructor asks a question and announces a time limit (1 to 3 minutes)
- Learners put their heads together to answer question
- Instructor calls a number, selects a group, and solicits a correct answer

Send a Problem (15 to 20 minutes)
- Learners each write a test review question on an index card
- The learner asks group members to answer
- If there is consensus about the right answer, it is written on the back
- If there are disagreements, the question is revised until all agree on an answer
- Groups forward questions to the next group

Concept Mapping (5 to 10 minutes)
- Instructor gives each group a large piece of poster paper
- Instructor gives each group member a different-colored marker
- Each group member adds a main concept
- Each member should then be free to add concepts and make connections
- Groups should share their maps and note how others connected concepts or developed subcategories

Structured Controversy (30 minutes to several hours)
- Instructor presents a controversy and provides material with supporting arguments for and against it or directs learners to acquire material to support their position
- Two learners prepare an argument for, and two learners prepare an argument against, the issue
- Each pair presents their arguments and evidence to the other pair; each pair must then switch sides and argue for the reverse side of the controversy, making the best arguments possible
- The group of four presents a consensus report on the issue

Groups

Many instructors have had uncomfortable personal and professional experiences working in groups. There are universal concerns about accountability and the time that group work takes. Instructors must have clearly defined objectives in mind in order to make productive use of learning time when they choose to have learners work in groups. Instructions about group work should be clearly stated.

Grades

Group projects should have both group and individual accountability identified. Frequently, instructors use self-evaluation and peer evaluation with a written log from each learner for validation of their scoring, which is based on the objectives of the project. There should also be an instructor evaluation of the group project. If possible, each member's contribution should also be evaluated. Thus a group project grade may have three or four scores, and members of the same group may have different grades based on their own, peer, and instructor evaluations.

Group Membership

Group membership should be determined by the instructor and not by learners. Group membership based on friendship tends to negate the opportunity to learn to work with people who are different from us. Adult learners may express unhappiness about not being with their friends. However, the long-term benefits of increased awareness of differences and improved social skills are adequate justification for instructor-made groups. Ideal group size is four but may vary from three to six members. Groups need to be small enough so that each member gets an opportunity to interact.

Instructors should have some easy and impartial method for determining group membership. One method might be to hand out a card to each learner as they enter the learning area from a shuffled deck of playing cards. Depending upon how large the group, use less than or more than one deck of cards. Groups of four can be formed by having learners with the same number or face card from each suit come together. Another advantage of using a deck of cards is that some exercises may require that a member from each small group will split off and join another group for part of the exercise. The split can be accomplished by using both card value and suit.

Group Rates

Specific roles should be identified and role assignments changed within groups so that all members have an opportunity to assume the different roles. Roles that should be considered are timekeeper, recorder, reporter, and monitor. The timekeeper is responsible for keeping the group on task and seeing that the work is completed within the stated time frames. The recorder is responsible for writing down the decision/thoughts of the group, and the reporter is responsible for offering a summary of the group's deliberations to the class at large. The monitor is responsible for ensuring that all members of the group participate in the discussion. It may prove helpful to have group roles briefly listed on four different-colored index cards that group members can pass around as they change roles. Several sets are needed so that each small group will have a full set. Additional roles are gatekeeper and praiser. The gatekeeper determines how much time each member can spend talking and the praiser acknowledges members' contributions.

Journals

Journals can be used to help learners clarify their thinking. Assignments can include writing objectives for clinical learning, self-evaluating clinical performance, writing a summary of an experience or observation, writing a critique of an article, or writing a focused article.

Objectives for Learning

- Objectives should reflect course content
- Objectives should be stated clearly and measurably
- Objectives should reflect one goal for each objective
- Learners should show reflection on progress to meet objectives

Self-evaluation of Clinical Performance

Learners may be directed to keep a clinical log. For reflection, the written appraisals should be kept in a bound journal, or if done on a computer, the hard copies should be submitted in a binder. Entries should be dated. Learners should address their performance, thoughts, and feelings regarding the clinical experience, and how the experience related to their course objectives. Broad guiding questions may be posed by faculty, but should not be considered exclusive. Yes/no answers to those questions are not sufficient to demonstrate critical thinking.

Sample Guiding Questions

- How did I identify physical, emotional, and learning needs of my client?
- How did I determine priority problems?
- What nursing skills did I perform?
- How did I demonstrate respect for my client as a person (cultural and spiritual values, dignity, privacy)?
- What did I do to manage care for the client?
- What were my strengths/weaknesses in the preparation for and in the performance of this clinical experience?
- How did these strengths/weaknesses affect my ability to perform client care?
- I plan to improve my performance by . . . .

Summaries

- The learner should be able to write a concise description of the observation or event

- The summary should be sequential, coherent, and gramatically correct
- The summary should be nonjudgmental

Critiques

Learners should be asked to address some or all of the following questions when preparing a 3- to 5-page paper on a topic. Topics should reflect course content and may be either learner-selected or instructor-selected. Learners may also be asked to compare and contrast two or more publications about a topic based on the same list of questions. Instructors may wish to add different questions depending on the focus of the course they are teaching.

- What point does the author make?
- What are the facts presented? Are there sufficient data in the article to support the author's ideas?
- Is the publication a summary, an overview, or a detailed analysis?
- Why did the author write the article?
- Was the author objective or biased?
- What was the source of the author's information (personal experience, experimentation, etc.)?
- What beliefs or attitudes does the author make apparent in the publication?
- What are the implications for you or your nursing career?
- What is your overall impression of the publication?

Focused Arguments

- Learners must take a position and offer arguments for or against an issue
- Learners may take the role of an imaginary figure and propose a solution to a problem from that person's imagined point of view

Graphic Organizers

In general, directions for concept mapping include the following: use colored paper wherever possible; use different-colored pens for different key concepts on the map; place the paper with the greatest width running from left to right (horizontal or landscape); place the central focus word in the center of the page and box it; use key words to represent ideas; use only one word per line; connect key words to the central focus word with lines; use pictures frequently; and finally, include the suggestions of *all* learners, regardless of their validity or veracity.

Clinical Correlation Mapping

- Create a problem list
- Draw the relationship between the problems (cause and effects)
- Associate pertinent laboratory and diagnostic tests related to each problem
- Specify your client's response to the identified problems
- Label appropriate nursing diagnoses
- Include NICs and NOCs

After completing the clinical correlation map (nursing process map), learners must be prepared to:

- Defend the choice of nursing diagnoses
- Explain the rationale for the priority nursing diagnoses
- Explain the rationale for the priority nursing interventions (NICs)
- Identify conclusions drawn from laboratory and diagnostic tests
- Defend the stated outcomes of care for the client (NOCs)
- Determine whether the stated outcomes for the client are being met

See the Appendix for further discussion.

Algorithms

Algorithms, also known as *decision trees,* are formed based on a dichotomous response at each problem level. Given the statement, "My activities today depend upon the weather. I will stay home if it rains, or I may go shopping or go to the beach." The decision is based on rain—yes or no—and then activities: stay home—yes or no—and, if no, then shopping—yes or no; if no, then go to the beach is the decision. A diagram of the decision tree might look like:

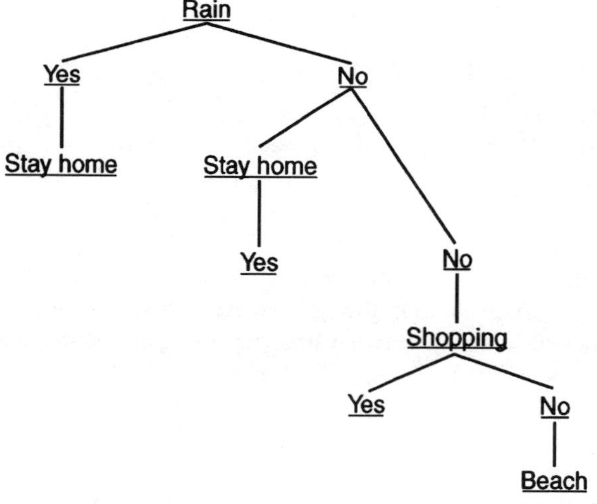

Algorithms are great aids to help learners examine the logical consequences of data, especially compare or contrast data set or an advantage versus disadvantage set. Both data sets permit the same either/or responses. Instructors can help learners to develop sequential thinking by asking them to construct algorithms. help learners to begin using algorithms by presenting them with an example such as the one shown. Discuss various ways that the algorithm might look—top down, branching horizontally, etc.

Sequence chains are a less rigid form of graphing events, but still require identification of what occurs first, next, and last. Many anatomy and physiology and pathophysiology books explain the dynamics of function or malfunction using a sequence or flow diagram. Again, help learners to use sequence chains by pointing out how to use them, give assignments that require them, and give feedback on learner use of the tools.

For many learners, being able to see several examples of graphic organizers is very helpful. In addition, working with others to construct and critique sequence chains or algorithms adds to the learner's sense of competency. Helping learners to organize knowledge for easy access and utilization requires that instructors call attention to thinking processes and tools. Graphic organizers are powerful vehicles to accomplish that task.

ANNOTATED BIBLIOGRAPHY

Concert Mapping

Baugh, N.G. and Mellott, K.G. (1998). Clinical concept mapping as preparation for student nurses' clinical experiences. *Journal of Nursing Education.* 37(6), 253-256.

Contains a very useful step-by-step set of instructions for students as well as illustrations for developing a clinical concept map. The instructions are clear, easy to set up, and easy to implement. The authors offer a short discussion on evaluation of student learning using their concept map.

Busan, T. (1993). *The Mind Map Book.* New York: Penguin Books.

The author presents the theory and mechanics of mind mapping. The book contains very clear step-by-step instructions for mind mapping with color plates and illustrations of mind maps. Suggestions are offered for projects appropriate for mind mapping. A must for anyone who is interested in using mind mapping.

Cannon, C.A. (1998). Path charting: A process and product for linking pathophysiological concepts. *Journal of Nursing Education.* 37(6), 257-259.

The author suggests that path charts can be used to help students visualize the interrelations among cause/risk factors, structural/functional alterations, and clinical manifestations. The article contains an illustration of the path chart and discusses directions to students to assist them to develop the charts. While the focus of the article was pathophysiology, the path chart can provide a useful first step for a clinical correlation map.

Daley, B.J. (1996). Concept maps: Linking nursing theory to clinical nursing practice. *The Journal of Continuing Education in Nursing.* 27(1), 17-27.

The article details the use of clinical concept maps to assess the level of student knowledge and preparation for clinical laboratory experiences. Several illustrations are included to show the comparison among six students. The author demonstrated that analysis of students concept maps can help faculty determine the students' ability to link theoretical knowledge in nursing and the sciences with clinical practice.

Irvine, L.M.C. (1995). Can concept mapping be used to promote meaningful learning in nurse education? *Journal of Advanced Nursing.* 21, 1175-1179.

The article defines concept mapping as "representing the individual's own interpretation of ideas in a diagrammatic form." A review of research on concept mapping and learning is presented. An example of a concept map on human circulation is included. The article includes an extensive bibliography on concept or mind mapping.

Kathol, D.D., Geiger, M.L., and Hartig, J.L. (1998). Clinical correlation map: A tool for linking theory and practice. *Nurse Educator.* 23(4), 31–34.

An excellent article with a case study and sample clinical correlation map. Six guidelines serve as foundation instructions for students in their preparation for developing a clinical correlation map. The students' visual representations assist instructors with the evaluation of student knowledge.

McTighe, J. (1991). Graphic organizers: Collaborative links to better thinking. In N. Davidson and T. Worsham, eds. *Enhancing Thinking Through Cooperative Learning.* New York: Teachers College Press.

The article has many illustrations of various types of graphic organizers and the types of assignments for which students might use the organizers. The author discusses how graphic organizers help students sequence and prioritize material.

Reynolds, A. (1994). Patho-flow diagramming: A strategy for critical thinking and clinical decision making. *Journal of Nursing Education.* 33(7), 333-336.

The article presents the theoretical bases for patho-flow diagramming. Several illustrations are included which show the associations that can be drawn from assessment data. The author describes how a curriculum can build students' ability to use patho-flow diagramming in stages. A brief discussion of grading the flowchart is included.

Rhooda, L.A. (1994). Effects of mind mapping on student achievement in a nursing research course. *Nurse Educator.* 19(6), 25-27.

The author describes a study that used mind mapping as a tool to improve student learning in a basic nursing research course. The conclusion was that mind mapping did improve student understanding and added an element of enjoyment to the class. The author offers suggestions to help faculty start using mind mapping and includes a useful illustration.

Wycoff, J. (1991). *Mind-mapping: Your Personal Guide to Exploring Creativity and Problem-solving.* New York: Berkley Books.

An exceptional resource for those interested in teaching mind mapping or concept mapping to students. The author leads readers through a progressive series of exercises that demonstrate the versatility and range of mind mapping. The book contains a wealth of illustrations and step-by-step instructions for various exercises.

Cooperative Learning

Johnson, D.W., Johnson, R.T., and Smith K.A. (1991). Cooperative learning: Increasing college faculty instructional productivity. ASHE-ERIC Higher Education Report No. 4. Washington, DC: The George Washington University, School of Education and Human Development.

Johnston, S., and Cooper, J. (1997). Quick-thinks: Active-thinking tasks in lecture classes and televised instruction. *Cooperative Learning and College Teaching.* 8(1), 2-6.

The article contains a discussion of cooperative learning techniques that are appropriate for televised instruction. In addition, eight instructional strategies are described and examples of their use are detailed. The publication contains a wealth of information on cooperative learning issues in higher education, and is a "must have" subscription for instructors interested in using cooperative learning in higher education.

Kagan, S. (1989). *Cooperative Learning Resources for Teachers.* San Juan Capistrano, CA: Resources for Teachers.

Practical how-to instructions for teachers interested in developing a wide variety of cooperative learning techniques. The author presents both theory and rationales for cooperative learning, including a discussion of group roles and responsibilities. In addition, the author presents an extensive array of cooperative learning structures such as pains-check, send-a-problem, numbered heads together, and others.

Kennedy, E.B. (1993). *An Investigation Using Independent, Collaborative Pairs, and Cooperative Group Practice for Teaching Cardiac Monitor Rhythm Strip Interpretation.* Ann Arbor, MI: UMI Dissertation Information Service.

This study investigated the effects of independent, collaborative pairs, and cooperative group practice on student accuracy, student practice time during lessons and performance time during skills testing, and the nature of student questions during skills testing. Associate degree nursing students are given the same instruction on how to analyze and interpret cardiac monitor rhythm strips followed by practice using one of the assigned practice modes. Cooperative group practice appeared to increase practice time and group performance time without sacrificing accuracy of performance.

Critical Thinking

Facione, N.C. and Facione, P.A. (1996). Externalizing the critical thinking in knowledge development and clinical judgment. *Nursing Outlook.* 44(3), 129-136.

The authors discuss the relationship of critical thinking to nursing. The article contains the consensus definition of critical thinking as well as a description of various critical thinking skills and subskills. The authors further delineate examples of a critical thinking evaluation rubric, directions for presenting a topic so that critical thinking is externalized, and a description of how to model critical thinking in the classroom and clinical setting.

Fonteyn, M.E. (1998). *Thinking Strategies for Nursing Practice.* 2nd ed. Gaithersburg, MD: Aspen Publishers, Inc.

Fuzard, B. (1989). *Innovative Teaching Strategies in Nursing.* 2nd ed. Gaithersburg, MD: Aspen Publishers, Inc.

Jacobs, P.M., Ott, B., Sullivan, B., Ulrich, Y., and Short, L. (1997). An approach to defining and operationalizing critical thinking. *Journal of Nursing Education.* 36(1), 19-22.

Marzano, R.J., Brandt, R.S., Hughes, C.S., Jones, B.F., Presseisen, B.Z., Rankin, S.C., and Suhor, C. (1988). *Dimensions of Thinking: A Framework for Curriculum and Instruction.* Alexandria, VA: Association for Supervision and Curriculum Development.

Whiteside, C. (1997). A model for teaching critical thinking in the clinical setting. *Dimensions of Critical Care Nursing.* 16(3), 152-162.

Internet Information

Harris, R. (1997). Evaluating internet research resources. http://www.virtualsalt.com/evalu8it.htm.

Lindell, C. (1998). The Internet medical and health information. http://www.med-legal.net

Sparks, S.M. and Rizzolo, M.A. (1998). World wide search tools. *Image: Journal of Nursing Scholarship.* 30(20), 167-171

Tillman, H.N. (2001). Evaluation quality on the net. http://www.hopetillman.com/findqual.html.

Journaling

Allen, D.G., Bowers, B., and Diekelmann, N. (1989). Writing to learn: A reconceptualization of thinking and writing in the nursing curriculum. *Journal of Nursing Education.* 28(1), 6-11.

The authors present a well-stated case for the use of focused writing assignments to develop thinking skills. The act of writing helps students to select and organize important information, which then functions to shape their understanding of the information. Writing is seen as interactive process, not a passive recording of events. A particularly useful discussion centers around the use of writing to help students transfer facts from one situation to another. Both curricular and classroom instructional suggestion are presented, and the advantages and disadvantages are described.

Atkins, S. and Murphy, K. (1993). Reflection: A review of the literature. *Journal of Advanced Nursing.* 18, 1188-1192.

The author presents a review of the literature describing reflective processes and the skills required to engage in reflective thinking. Among the skills identified are self-awareness, critical analysis, and evaluation.

Bratt, M.M. (1998). Reflective journaling: Fostering learning in clinical experiences. *Dean's Notes.* 20(1), 1-3.

The reflective thinking process is described in detail. Elements such as association, integration, validation, and appropriation are discussed as they apply to reflection. The act of putting thoughts down on paper improves student skills of interpretation, analysis, and synthesis. The importance of time to think and to write both from student and faculty perspectives is discussed.

Gartner, A., Latham, G., and Merritt, S. (1998). *The Power of Narrative: Transcending Disciplines.* http://ultiBASE.rmit.edu.au/develop/Articles/gartnl.html.

Hammer, D. (1997). The interactive journal: Creating a learning space. *PS: Political Science & Politics.* 30(1), 70-74.

Hughes, H.W., Kooy, M., and Kaneevsky, L. (1997). Dialogic reflection and journaling. *The Clearinghouse.* 70(4), 187-190.

McConchie, R. (1998). Journaling and reflection. http://chchpoly.ac.nz/polyinfo/healthsc/Journeys%20vol%203/mcconchi.htm.

Soldner, L.B. (1997). Self-assessment and the reflective reader. *Journal of College Reading and Learning.* 28(1), 5-12.

Teaching-Learning

Anderson, C.A. (1996) Teaching is not feeding. *Nursing Outlook.* 14(6), 257-258

This article written by the journal's editor briefly reviews how faculty supply students with many tools, such as large course syllabi, that do not stimulate the students to seek out information or employ critical thinking skills. Her main point is that we "feed" students instead of facilitating their learning using the principles of adult education.

Barr, R. and Tagg, J. (1995). From teaching to learning: A new paradigm for undergraduate education. *Change.* (Nov/Dec) 13-25.

The authors provide an innovative approach to the teaching-learning process by comparing a focus on teaching with a focus on learning. When faculty and educational institutions approach their students in a learning mode, they can be assured that students do learn. If they approach students in a teaching mode, students often do not learn. The chart in the article comparing these two approaches is extremely thought-provoking and not limited to undergraduate education.

CONTENTS

TRANSPARENCY MASTERS

UNIT 1 HEALTH PROMOTION AND ILLNESS ■ Core Concepts Grid

Critical Thinking in the Role of the Medical-Surgical Nurse	Community-Based Care	Introduction to Managed Care and Case Management	Introduction to Complementary and Alternative Therapies	Health Care of Older Adults
• **Definitions of health** • **Health promotion and protection** • **Roles** • **Teaching/learning process** • **Concept of caring** • **Practice settings** • **Nursing process**	• **Ambulatory care** • **Home care** • **Nursing home care** • **Subacute care** • **Rehabilitative care**	• **Purpose** Types • **Role of the nurse** • **Focus on outcomes** • **Case management** • **Role of case manager** • **Clinical pathways**	• **Spirituality and religion** • **Relaxation** • **Imagery** • **Music** • **Touch** • **Laughter/humor** • **Herbalism** • **Progressive muscle relaxation** • **Aromatherapy**	• **Subgroups of older adults** • **Health issues** Health promotion Nutritional needs Accidents Drug use/misuse Mental health Neglect/abuse • **Economic issues** Income Housing Other resources • **Role of gerontologic nurse**

Unit 1 (Chapters 1-5)

Health Promotion and Illness

Learning Plan

Chapter 1: *Critical Thinking in the Role of the Medical-Surgical Nurse*

Learning Outcomes	Learning Activities	Supplemental Resources
After studying this chapter, the student should be able to: 1. Compare and contrast common definitions of health. 2. Explain why some populations are more likely to experience health problems than others. 3. Differentiate the three levels of illness prevention and provide at least one example of each level. 4. Explain the purpose of Healthy People 2010. 5. Identify the major roles of the medical-surgical nurse. 6. Explain the relationship between critical thinking and evidence-based practice. 7. Describe best practice interventions for client education. 8. Describe typical health care settings in which medical-surgical nursing is practiced. 9. Identify the key components of a nursing assessment. 10. Describe the difference between a nursing diagnosis and a collaborative problem. 11. Formulate expected outcomes based on data analysis. 12. Identify best practice interventions for clinical documentation.	**Think-pair-share (3-5 min)** Have learners share a brief personal definition of "health." Compare commonalities and differences. List methods to promote health and prevent illness for clients in a hospital setting; identify each method as primary, secondary, or tertiary. Identify similarities and differences between nursing practice in acute care and that in long-term care. For the client used in the journalizing exercise above, develop expected outcomes for each nursing diagnosis and collaborative problem. List the similarities and differences between a nursing care plan and an interdisciplinary plan of care. What are the advantages of using a clinical pathway as the plan of care? **Pairs check (15-20 min)** Have learners take a nursing history on each other and document it using any nursing database. **Concept mapping (10-15 min)** Have learners form groups of 4 or 5; map the major roles of the medical-surgical nurse in acute care, long-term care, ambulatory care, and home care. Have one learner report the group's map and compare with others. **Journaling (15-20 min)** Have learners record their own health promotion/illness prevention practices for 1 week. Reflect on what practices could be improved, if any. Using any client's nursing database, identify at least two actual or potential nursing diagnoses and at least two collaborative problems.	**Internet resources** Healthy People http://web.health.gov/healthypeople/ Upstate University: CEBP Home page http://www.upstate.edu/cebp/index.htm Centre for Evidence Based Nursing http://www.york.ac.uk/depts/hstd/centres/evidence/acute4.htm Community-Based Care: A Nursing Education Project http://www.southalabama.edu/nursing/fuld/ **Community resources** Invite a nurse from the local holistic nurses' group to discuss his or her practice. Visit an Integrative Medicine Department of a health care system or hospital. Have a nurse from a local Health Department visit and discuss specific health initiatives that are provided to the community (e.g., free or low-cost blood pressure/cholesterol monitoring).

Chapter 2: *Community-Based Care*		
Learning Outcomes	**Learning Activities**	**Supplemental Resources**
After studying this chapter, the student should be able to: 1. Explain the primary purpose of ambulatory care. 2. Discuss the growth of home care in the United States. 3. Describe the role of the nurse in home care. 4. Identify examples of interventions for which Medicare pays in-home care. 5. Compare and contrast the common types of nursing homes. 6. Describe the term *subacute care*.	**Think-pair-share (3-5 min)** List the types of clients typically admitted to subacute care units. List the types of clients typically requiring home care. Identify the types of clients typically requiring nursing home placement. Why are clients in nursing homes referred to as "residents"? **Journaling (10-15 min)** Have the learner describe successful health teaching for a client being discharged from the hospital to home.	**Internet resources** Homecare Online http://www.nahc.org/ Directory of Home Care Resources http://www.providerconsult.com/resources/entry.htm **Community resources** Invite a panel of nursing home, home care, ambulatory care, and acute care nurses to discuss why they chose to work in their settings. Visit a subacute care unit and provide care as assigned. Care for residents on a skilled unit of a nursing home. Assist in the care of clients in the home care setting. Assist in the care of clients in ambulatory care (outpatient clinics, HMOs, or physicians' offices).

Chapter 3: *Introduction to Managed Care and Case Management*		
Learning Outcomes	**Learning Activities**	**Supplemental Resources**
After studying this chapter, the student should be able to: 1. Explain the primary purpose of managed health care. 2. Contrast the fee-for-service and capitated reimbursement systems. 3. Describe the process of case management. 4. Identify at least three certifications for case managers.	**Think-pair-share (3-5 min)** Compare the nursing process with the case management process. Identify ways for lay caregivers to manage their stress. **Journaling (10-15 min)** Have learners recall two clients they have cared for who would benefit from case management referral; state how a case manager would be helpful in each case. **Concept mapping (5-10 min)** Map the case management process.	**Internet resource** The Case Management Society of America http://www.cmsa.org/ **Community resources** Spend a day with a case manager in any health care setting, including occupational health, acute care, rehabilitation, home care, or long term care to observe his or her role. Invite a case manager from the local hospital to discuss his or her role and relationship with the nursing staff.

		Invite a case manager from a managed care company to discuss telephonic case management and how it is different from hospital case management.

Chapter 4: *Introduction to Complementary and Alternative Therapies*

Learning Outcomes	Learning Activities	Supplemental Resources
After studying this chapter, the student should be able to: 1. Describe selected low-risk complementary and alternative therapies that nurses can use with their clients in a variety of health care settings. 2. Identify at least one purpose for each selected complementary and alternative therapy. 3. Discuss the implications of complementary and alternative therapies for health care professionals.	**Pairs check (5-10 min)** For any client cared for, have learners write a narrative nursing note, then use the FOCUS format to rewrite the same information, keeping the legal aspects of documentation in mind. **Journaling (10-15 min)** Interview a client who has had success using acupuncture or biofeedback therapy to resolve a health problem.	**Internet resources** American Holistic Nurses Association http://www.ahna.org/ American Massage Therapy Association http://www.amtamassage.org/ Complementary Therapies http://www.wholenurse.com/ Healing Touch International http://www.healingtouch.net/ Nurses Certification Program in Interactive Imagery http://imageryrn.com/ **Community resources** Invite a massage therapist or music therapist to discuss the benefits of these therapies. Visit a biofeedback laboratory to observe the various reasons why biofeedback is used. Invite a risk manager, paralegal expert, or nurse attorney to discuss cases where medical-surgical nurses have been sued for malpractice based on inadequate documentation.

Chapter 5: *Health Care of Older Adults*

Learning Outcomes	Learning Activities	Supplemental Resources
After studying this chapter, the student should be able to: 1. Identify four subgroups of older adults. 2. Describe nursing interventions for relocation stress syndrome. 3. Discuss common health issues that may concern older adults. 4. Explain why older adults are often at high risk for falls. 5. State common interventions for older clients at high risk for falls. 6. Describe the nursing care required for clients who are restrained. 7. Explain the effects of drugs on the older adult. 8. Compare and contrast delirium and dementia. 9. Interpret the signs and symptoms of elder neglect or abuse. 10. Discuss potential economic issues for older adults. 11. Describe government and community resources that are available for older adults.	**Think-pair-share (3-5 min)** Complete TM 5-1 prior to class; discuss and compare answers. Complete TM 5-2 prior to class; discuss and compare answers. List the factors that can positively or negatively affect a client's ability to learn. List community services that are available for the elderly. What are the advantages and disadvantages of physical restraints, such as a vest, for an elderly client? What are the dangers of chemical restraints, especially when given to the elderly? Develop a brief teaching-learning plan for any client with a new medical diagnosis. Identify resources that an elderly client having a total knee replacement will need at home. **Pairs check (5-10 min)** Practice applying and tying a vest restraint using a quick-release knot. **Concept mapping (10-15 min)** Map the effect of medications on the elderly; include both physiologic and psychosocial aspects. Map the factors that place hospitalized elderly at risk for falls. **Journaling (10-15 min)** Select at least one physiologic and one psychosocial theory of aging and defend it as a viable theory. **Team concept mapping (10-15 min)** Have learners map the effects of aging on body image.	**Transparency masters** TM 5-1 Comparison of young, middle, and late adulthood TM 5-2 Comparison of the three D's: Delirium, dementia, and depression **Internet resources** A Place for Mom.com http://www.aplaceformom.com/ Ageless Design: Smarter, Safer Living for Seniors http://www.agelessdesign.com/alz.htm **Community resources** Visit a Senior Citizens' Center to practice interviewing skills and observe normal physiologic and psychosocial changes associated with aging. Invite the local Office on Aging ombudsman to discuss his or her role, as well as the local community services available for the elderly. Spend part of a day with a community service, such as Meals on Wheels or Senior Ride. Invite a clinical pharmacist or gerontology clinical nurse specialist to discuss medication usage in the elderly client and nursing implications. Spend a day with a gerontological or medical-surgical clinical nurse specialist to observe his or her role. Invite a family member who is caring for a loved one with Alzheimer's disease to discuss a typical day as a caregiver and how he or she manages stress.

TM 5-1

COMPARISON OF YOUNG, MIDDLE, AND LATE ADULTHOOD

	Young Adulthood	**Middle Adulthood**	**Late Adulthood**
Physical changes			
Psychosocial changes			
Common accidents/ illnesses			
Nursing implications for health promotion			

TM 5-2

COMPARISON OF THE THREE Ds: DELIRIUM, DEMENTIA, AND DEPRESSION

	Delirium	**Dementia**	**Depression**
Etiology/risk factors			
Clinical manifestations/ behaviors			
Interdisciplinary management			

UNIT 2 BIOPSYCHOSOCIAL CONCEPTS RELATED TO HEALTH CARE ■ Core Concepts Grid

Concepts	Assessment	Assessment	Concepts
• **Culture** Definition Cultural competence Assessment Cultural care plan Religion Folk medicine Pain Ethics • **Pain** Theories of pain Types of pain Addiction Dependence Tolerance Placebos • **Substance abuse** Stimulants Hallucinogens Depressants Narcotics Inhalants Steroids • **End-of-life care** Goals Hospice care Death Postmortem care Euthanasia • **Rehabilitation** Settings Team	• **Pain** Site/location Intensity Quality/chronology Nonverbal indicators of pain Vital signs Anxiety Sweating Restlessness Confusion • **Substance abuse** Hallucinations Seizures Cardiac dysrhythmias Dilated pupils Vital sign changes Tremors Nausea/vomiting Abdominal cramps Mental health disorders Visual disturbances Euphoria Relaxation Sexual arousal Poor attention and memory • **End-of-life care** Lethargy Decreased level of consciousness (LOC) Discomfort or pain Dyspnea Agitation Nausea/vomiting Dysphagia • **Rehabilitation** Body system assessment Functional assessment Psychosocial assessment Vocational assessment	• **Pain** Monitoring pain Cutaneous stimulation Distraction Acupuncture Imagery Transcutaneous electrical nerve stimulation (TENS) Heat/cold Touch • **Substance abuse** Health teaching Avoidance Rehabilitation Symptom management • **End-of-life care** Oxygen Oral hygiene Alternative drug routes Positioning Rest Energy conservation Foley catheter Enema Physical support Presence Being realistic Promoting spirituality Referral to bereavement services Health teaching • **Rehabilitation** Transfers Gait training Prevention of complications of immobility Assistive/adaptive devices Energy conservation Skin care Bladder and bowel training Community-based care	• **Pain** Nonopioid drugs Opioid analgesics Tricyclic antidepressants Other adjunctive drugs • **End-of-life care** Opioids in varying routes Diuretics Bronchodilators Corticosteroids Antibiotics Anticholinergics Sedatives Antianxiety drugs Barbiturates • **Rehabilitation** Cholinergics Rectal suppositories

Unit 2 (Chapters 6-10)

Biopsychosocial Concepts Related to Health Care

Learning Plan

Chapter 6: *Cultural Aspect of Health*

Learning Outcomes	Learning Activities	Supplemental Resources
After studying this chapter, the student should be able to: 1. Define cultural competence, culture, and subculture. 2. Explain the purpose of Healthy People 2010 as it relates to cultural groups. 3. Describe the three methods for assessing the culture of a client or group. 4. Identify two subcultures that have often been neglected. 5. Discuss specific cultural practices – religion, nutrition and folk medicine – that the nurse should consider when assessing a client's culture.	**Pairs check (10-15 min)** Have learners perform a cultural assessment on each other; document three findings that could impact nursing care (e.g., diet restrictions). **Think-pair-share (3-5 min)** Discuss how disease and illness can be affected by one's culture. Identify how culture, especially religion, affects how an individual copes with loss and death. **Concept mapping (10-15 min)** Map the relationship between culture and acute/chronic illness.	**Internet resources** Pro-Cultura, Inc. http://www.procultura.org/ Healthy People http://web.health.gov/healthypeople/ **Community resources** Invite individuals from different cultures to attend a class discussion – include beliefs about religion, diet, and medicine/healing. Have class members with differing cultural backgrounds join in the discussion. As a focus, discuss the adaptations that nurses must make in providing care to clients with diverse cultural beliefs.

Chapter 7: *Pain: The Fifth Vital Sign*

Learning Outcomes	Learning Activities	Supplemental Resources
After studying this chapter, the student should be able to: 1. Define the concept of pain. 2. Describe briefly the gate control theory to explain the relationship between pain and emotion. 3. Explain the role of neuromodulators in the experience of pain. 4. Identify variables that influence a client's perception of pain.	**Think-pair-share (3-5 min)** Have learners complete TM 7-1 prior to class; compare answers. Have learners complete TM 7-2 prior to class; compare answers. Have learners perform a pain assessment on any hospitalized or home care client using any pain assessment tool. Discuss the etiology and pathophysiology of phantom limb pain following an amputation.	**Transparency masters** TM 7-1 Comparison of acute, chronic malignant, and chronic nonmalignant pain TM 7-2 Common analgesics used for pain **Internet resources** American Academy of Pain Management http://www.aapainmanage.org/

5. Discuss the attitudes and knowledge of nurses, physicians, and clients regarding pain assessment and management. 6. Compare and contrast the characteristics of the major types of pain. 7. Describe the components of a comprehensive pain assessment. 8. Analyze assessment data to formulate nursing diagnoses for the client experiencing pain. 9. Plan nursing care for the client experiencing acute pain. 10. Differentiate commonly used drugs for acute pain and chronic pain. 11. Describe the nursing implications associated with drug therapy for clients with acute pain or chronic pain. 12. Identify special considerations for older adults related to pain assessment and management. 13. Discuss complementary and alternative therapies for clients experiencing pain. 14. Develop a teaching/learning plan for managing pain as part of community-based care for clients experiencing pain.	**Concept mapping (10-15 min)** Map the concepts of acute and chronic pain. **Send a problem (10-15 min)** Have learners write a test review question on the use of TENS devices to manage pain. **Structured controversy (10-15 min)** Should complementary therapies be used to manage pain? **Structured controversy (15-20 min)** Should marijuana be legalized for cancer pain control?	pain.com http://www.pain.com/ **Community resources** Invite an expert in pain management to demonstrate relaxation and other techniques for pain control. Visit a pain clinic and determine its function; participate in the care of clients with chronic pain. Visit an Integrative Medicine department of a health care system to determine what modalities are used for pain control. Explore a TENS unit and how it is applied. Interview an individual who is experiencing a problem with chronic pain. Document methods used (past and present) to control the pain.

Chapter 8: *Substance Abuse*

Learning Outcomes	Learning Activities	Supplemental Resources
After studying this chapter, the student should be able to: 1. Discuss substance abuse as a major health problem in the United States. 2. Explain the effects of substance abuse on the mental and physical health of individuals and society. 3. Describe the relationship between stress and substance abuse. 4. Identify assessment findings associated with the use of stimulants, hallucinogens, depressants, opioids, inhalants, and steroids.	**Think-pair-share (3-5 min)** Discuss methods to effectively assess substance abuse in a hospitalized client. List several ways to effectively communicate with a client who is suspected of abusing a substance. **Concept mapping (10-15 min)** Map the concepts of two types of substance abuse.	**Internet resources** Substance Abuse and Addiction Information Support http://www.supportpilot.com/substance.html SAMHSA's National Clearinghouse for Alcohol and Drug Information http://www.health.org/ **Community resources** Attend an Alcoholics Anonymous (AA) meeting and note the interactions among group members.

5. Discuss priorities for care of clients who have or are experiencing substance abuse. 6. Identify signs and symptoms of alcohol with-drawal.	**Structured controversy (15-20 min)** Should families and friends of abusing clients be "con-frontational" with the abuser? If so, why? If not, why?	Attend an ALANON meeting and note the interactions of those who live with alcoholics. Explore programs for smoking cessation in your com-munity. Inquire about the success rates of these pro-grams. Have a local law enforcement officer speak to your nursing class about the substance abuse problems prevalent in your community. Discuss methods to control these problems.

Chapter 9: *End-of-Life Care*

Learning Outcomes	Learning Activities	Supplemental Resources
After studying this chapter, the student should be able to: 1. Explain the goals of end-of-life care. 2. Describe the hospice concept. 3. Interpret the common physical and emotional signs of impending death. 4. Identify interventions for managing symptoms of distress at end of life. 5. Describe postmortem care. 6. Compare active euthanasia and passive euthanasia.	**Think-pair-share (3-5 min)** Complete TM 9-1 prior to class; compare answers. **Structured controversy (15-20 min)** Should tube feeding be removed upon family request for a client in a persistent vegetative state (PVS)? Should passive euthanasia be legalized in the United States? **Send a problem (10-15 min)** Have learners write a test review question on decision-making models for ethical dilemmas in medical-surgical nursing practice. Have learners write a test review question on types of euthanasia.	**Transparency master** TM 9-1 Ethical issues in medical-surgical nursing **Internet resources** Choice in Dying http://www.choices.org/ Funeral and Memorial Societies of America http://www.funerals.org/ Hospice Association of America http://www.nahc.org/ **Community resources** Invite a bereavement counselor to describe his or her role. Attend a bereavement support group meeting.

	Journaling (10-15 min) Have learners describe their experience doing hospice visits; include feelings about caring for a client who is dying. Manage care for a dying client. **Structured controversy (15-20 min)** Should a client be allowed to refuse all food and water with the intent of accelerating his or her own death? **Numbered heads together (3-5 min)** What are the advantages and disadvantages of the living will and durable power of attorney for health care? Are verbal advance directives acceptable in the absence of written advance directives?	Invite a paralegal assistant or nurse attorney to discuss written and verbal advance directives. Invite a hospice nurse to discuss his or her role in providing comfort measures for terminal clients. Go on visits with a hospice nurse and participate in care of at least one client.

Chapter 10: *Rehabilitation Concepts for Acute and Chronic Problems*

Learning Outcomes	Learning Activities	Supplemental Resources
After studying this chapter, the student should be able to: 1. Differentiate between impairment, disability, and handicap. 2. Identify the roles of each member of the interdisciplinary rehabilitation team. 3. Interpret physical assessment findings for the client in a rehabilitation program. 4. Describe the major components of a functional assessment. 5. Prioritize nursing care for the client in a rehabilitation program. 6. Develop a teaching plan for the rehabilitation client at risk for complications of impaired physical mobility. 7. Assess client outcomes of the interdisciplinary rehabilitation program. 8. Explain the primary concerns for clients being discharged to home after rehabilitation.	**Think-pair-share (3-5 min)** Have learners perform a functional assessment on any client using any acceptable tool. List common complications of immobility associated with clients who have a spinal cord injury. List risk factors that place clients who are being rehabilitated at high risk for pressure ulcer development. List nursing interventions that help prevent pressure ulcers. Develop a care plan for bladder and bowel training for a client with a low level paraplegia (lower motor neuron lesion). **Pairs check (5-10 min)** Position each other while supine and sitting to prevent pressure on bony prominences. Have learners simulate having a left-sided stroke; practice transfer techniques from the bed to the chair and vice versa.	**Internet resources** The Simon Foundation for Continence http://www.simonfoundation.org/ National Association for Continence http://www.nafc.org/ American Paralysis Association http://www.apacure.com/ **Community resources** Invite a counselor from a rehabilitation setting to discuss his or her role. Visit several types of rehabilitation settings, including a skilled nursing facility and a freestanding rehabilitation center; focus on the role of each health team member. Invite a rehabilitation case manager to discuss continuum of care issues for the disabled client.

	For the above simulation, have learners assist each other with ambulation using a cane and gait belt. Have learners simulate paraplegia and quadriplegia: practice transfers using sliding board and "bear-hug" techniques. **Journaling (10 min)** Care for a client in the home who is receiving rehabilitation services (PT, OT, SLP); record the role(s) of each of these health team members. Record experiences from visits to the community, including how nurses can use these resources for their clients (e.g., visit to a rehabilitation unit or pain clinic). Participate in interdisciplinary care for the client in a rehabilitation setting (e.g., multiple sclerosis, spinal cord injury, stroke). **Journaling (10-15 min)** Interview any client with a chronic illness who is disabled; record his or her coping strategies and interaction with society. **Structured controversy (10-15 min)** Should government monies be used for rehabilitation of clients who refused to wear seat belts or wear motorcycle helmets? At what age should clients no longer be considered as candidates for rehabilitation?	Invite a client who has had a mastectomy, ostomy, or amputation to discuss body image changes and coping mechanisms. Attend an interdisciplinary team meeting in a rehabilitation setting. Visit an "apartment" in a rehabilitation setting and observe how the occupational therapist helps the client with activities of daily living (ADL) rehabilitation.

TM 7-1

COMPARISON OF ACUTE, CHRONIC MALIGNANT, AND CHRONIC NONMALIGNANT PAIN

	Acute Pain	**Chronic Malignant Pain**	**Chronic Nonmalignant Pain**
Definition/ description			
Clinical manifestations/ characteristics			
Commonly used drug therapy			
Nonpharma-cologic interventions			

TM 7-2

COMMON ANALGESICS USED FOR PAIN

	Over-the-Counter (OTC) Drugs	**Prescription NSAIDs**	**Opioid Analgesics**
Examples of drugs			
Indications/uses			
Side/adverse effects			
Nursing considerations/ interventions			

TM 9-1

ETHICAL ISSUES IN MEDICAL-SURGICAL NURSING

List examples of each ethical issue/dilemma. Be prepared to discuss with your peers.

Issue	**Example**
Futility	
Quality of life	
Palliative care	
Legal competency	
Placebo administration	
Restraints	
Confidentiality	
Unethical professional conduct	
Verbal advance directive	
Living will	
Durable power of attorney for health care	

UNIT 3

MANAGEMENT OF CLIENTS WITH FLUID, ELECTROLYTE, AND ACID-BASE IMBALANCES

■ Core Concepts Grid

Anatomy	Physiology	Pathophysiology	History	Physical Exam	Diagnostic Tests	Interventions	Pharmacology
• **Body fluid** Intercellular Extracellular Intravascular Interstitial • **Lungs** • **Heart/vessels** • **Kidney**	• **Filtration** • **Osmosis** • **Diffusion** • **Active transport** • **Hydrostatic pressure** • **Tonicity** Isotonic Hypotonic Hypertonic • **Third-space fluids** • **Transport medium** • **Protection** • **Metabolism** • **Regulatory mechanisms for fluid-electrolyte balance** • **Regulatory mechanisms for acid-base balance**	• **Overhydration** • **Dehydration** Isotonic Hypertonic Hypotonic • **Solute excess** • **Solute deficit** • **Metabolic acidosis/ alkalosis** • **Respiratory acidosis/ alkalosis**	• **Client history** Anorexia Fatigue Headache Nausea/ vomiting Diarrhea Weakness Cramping Thirst Fever	• **Skin** Color/moisture Turgor • **Weight** • **Urine output** • **Vital signs** • **Breath sounds** • **Muscle weakness** • **Central nervous system** Mental status Hyperreflexia Tetany Chvostek's sign Trousseau's sign • **Cardiovascular system** Dysrhythmias Decreased cardiac output	• **Serum levels** Sodium Potassium Calcium Phosphorus Magnesium • **Urine tests** pH Specific gravity • **Blood urea nitrogen** • **Arterial blood gases** pH Pao_2 $Paco_2$ HCO_3 • **Anion gap** • **Hemoglobin/ hematocrit**	• **Oral rehydration** • **Therapeutic diets** • **Blood gas interpretation** • **Semi-Fowler's position** • **Respiratory** Oxygen Turn, cough, deep breathe Incentive spirometry • **Oral hygiene** • **Rest** • **Infusion therapy** Peripheral intravenous therapy Central intravenous therapy • **Health teaching**	• **Diuretics** • **Crystalloid/ colloid fluid replacement** • **Electrolyte replacement** • **Bronchodilators** • **Anti-inflammatory drugs** • **Antibiotics** • **Antidiarrheals** • **Kayexelate**

Unit 3 (Chapters 11-16)

Management of Clients with Fluid, Electrolyte, and Acid-Base Imbalances

Learning Plan

Chapter 11: *Fluid and Electrolyte Balance*

Learning Outcomes	Learning Activities	Supplemental Resources
After studying this chapter, the student should be able to: 1. Explain why women and older adults have less total body water than do men and younger adults. 2. Interpret whether a client's serum electrolyte values are normal, elevated, or low. 3. Describe the expected blood volume and osmolarity responses when isotonic, hypertonic, or hypotonic intravenous fluids are infused. 4. Explain the relationships between antidiuretic hormone, urine output volume, and osmolarity. 5. Analyze a client's hydration status on the basis of physical assessment findings. 6. Evaluate a client's food choices for compliance with a low-sodium diet.	**Think-pair-share (3-5 min)** Complete TM 11-1 prior to class; compare answers. List the most commonly used IV fluids and color-code them as isotonic, hypertonic, or hypertonic. Determine a common condition that would require using an isotonic, hypotonic, or hypertonic IV infusion. **Concept mapping (10-15 min)** Have learners draw/copy human figures at various developmental ages and show the percentages of "total body water" at each age. Have learners map the concept of edema. **Pairs check (10-15 min)** Make flash cards of the most common electrolyte values and take turns quizzing until all are memorized. Role-play checking for the common signs and symptoms of overhydration and dehydration. Have learners maintain a food diary for 24 hours—keeping account of the amount of sodium consumed. Make a list of the high and low sodium items that learners report.	**Transparency master** TM 11-1 Laboratory findings in the client with dehydration **Internet resources** (See lists in other units for specific diseases; e.g., American Heart Association for cardiac disorders.) **Community resources** Invite an infusion therapy nurse to discuss his or her role in caring for clients with fluid and electrolyte imbalances.

Chapter 12: *Interventions for Clients with Fluid Imbalances*

Learning Outcomes	Learning Activities	Supplemental Resources
After studying this chapter, the student should be able to: 1. Identify clients at risk for fluid imbalances. 2. Use laboratory data and clinical manifestations to determine the presence of fluid imbalance.	**Think-pair-share (3-5 min)** Complete TM 12-1 prior to class; compare answers. List changes in fluid, electrolyte, and acid-base balance associated with aging. Discuss methods that are successful in getting older adults to drink fluids.	**Transparency master** TM 12-1 Comparison of fluid deficit and fluid overload **Internet resources** Edema and Water Retention http://www.thecountrydoctor.com/edema.htm

3. Apply appropriate nursing techniques to promote comfort and safety in the client with dehydration. 4. Prioritize nursing care for the client with fluid imbalance. 5. Develop a teaching plan to prevent dehydration in the older client at continuing risk for fluid loss. 6. Analyze changes in clinical manifestations to determine the effectiveness of therapy for the client with fluid imbalance.	**Pairs check (10-15 min)** Write a focused "fluid volume" care plan for a client with: • Acute dehydration • Acute overhydration Prioritize nursing interventions. **Team concept mapping (10-15 min)** Have learners map the concept of third spacing, including ascites as an example.	Water and Sodium Metabolism http://www.merck.com/pubs/mmanual/section2/chapter12/12b.htm **Community resources** Visit a local Senior Center and survey members about their "fluid intake" habits. Be prepared to do some "on the spot" teaching about helping them determine when they might be dehydrated.

Chapter 13: *Interventions for Clients with Electrolyte Imbalances*

Learning Outcomes	Learning Activities	Supplemental Resources
After studying this chapter, the student should be able to: 1. Identify clients at risk for imbalances of potassium. 2. Use laboratory data and clinical manifestations to determine the presence of potassium imbalance. 3. Prioritize nursing care for the client with potassium imbalance. 4. Develop a teaching plan to prevent deficiencies or excesses of potassium in the older adult client at risk for potassium imbalance. 5. Analyze changes in clinical manifestations to determine the effectiveness of therapy for the client with potassium imbalance. 6. Identify clients at risk for imbalances of sodium. 7. Use laboratory data and clinical manifestations to determine the presence of sodium imbalance. 8. Prioritize nursing care for the client with sodium imbalance. 9. Develop a teaching plan to prevent deficiencies or excesses of sodium in the older adult client at risk for sodium imbalance.	**Think-pair-share (3-5 min)** What fluid and electrolyte replacements do clients receive during and after surgery? Why? How do diuretics work in the management of clients with fluid overload? What side/adverse effects are common with most diuretics? How are loop diuretics different from potassium-sparing diuretics? What assessment findings may be evident in clients experiencing hyperkalemia? How does hypercalcemia occur in clients with advanced cancer? What is the treatment for clients experiencing hypernatremia? What is the best indicator of fluid balance in the body? **Concept mapping (10-15 min)** Make a chart with the headings of: • Potassium • Sodium • Calcium List normal values and what an ↑ or a ↓ in each will mean to the client—subjectively and objectively. Color-code or highlight critical signs and symptoms.	**Internet resources** Potassium Imbalance http://www.merck.com/pubs/mmanual/section2/chapter12/12c.htm Rheumatoid Arthritis Treatment by Potassium http://members.tripod.com/~charles_W/arthritis.html Salt-Free Life: A Guide to Sodium-Free Cuisine http://www.saltfree.com/ Calcium – Nutritional Health Information http://www.naturalways.com/calciumResearch.htm **Community resources** Invite a clinical pharmacist to discuss the dangers of IV potassium. Have an Intensivist speak to the class about the importance of electrolyte balance—with particular emphasis on potassium, sodium, and calcium.

10. Analyze changes in clinical manifestations to determine the effectiveness of therapy for the client with sodium imbalance. 11. Identify clients at risk for imbalances of calcium. 12. Use laboratory data and clinical manifestations to determine the presence of calcium imbalance. 13. Prioritize nursing care for the client with calcium imbalance. 14. Develop a teaching plan to prevent deficiencies or excesses of calcium in the older adult client at risk for calcium imbalance. 15. Analyze changes in clinical manifestations to determine the effectiveness of therapy for the client with calcium imbalance.	**Pairs check (10-15 min)** In the lab and/or in a clinical setting, add potassium chloride (KCl) to an IV solution. Properly label the bag and calculate a safe flow rate.	

Chapter 14: *Infusion Therapy*

Learning Outcomes	Learning Activities	Supplemental Resources
After studying this chapter, the student should be able to: 1. Explain the purpose of infusion filters. 2. Explain the primary advantage of needleless infusion systems. 3. Compare and contrast the use of controllers and pumps. 4. Identify important considerations when placing a venous access device (VAD). 5. Determine special needs of older adults who receive intravenous (IV) therapy. 6. Describe the major difference between nontunneled and tunneled central VADs. 7. Describe how a peripherally inserted central catheter differs from central lines. 8. Compare and contrast the major complications of peripheral and central IV therapy.	**Think-pair-share (3-5 min)** Identify common complications of IV therapy and how they can be prevented. List special considerations for elderly clients receiving IV therapy. **Pairs check (10-15 min)** Have learners demonstrate changing peripheral and central line dressings. Have learners demonstrate how to use a needleless IV tubing system. Have learners practice starting a peripheral IV using an arm model.	**Internet resources** Infusion Nurses Society—Webpage http://www.ins1.org/ **Community resources** Visit an infusion center and note the role of the infusion therapy nurse. Have learners practice using electronic infusion pumps in the hospital, home, or nursing home setting. Note differences in ambulatory pumps when compared with those used in hospitals.

9. Identify the most common use for intra-arterial therapy. 10. Describe the nursing care of a client receiving hypodermoclysis. 11. Explain the indications for epidural and intrathecal therapies.		

Chapter 15: *Acid-Base Balance*

Learning Outcomes	Learning Activities	Supplemental Resources
After studying this chapter, the student should be able to: 1. Describe the relationship between hydrogen ion concentration and pH. 2. Explain the role of bicarbonate in the blood. 3. Explain the concept of compensation. 4. Compare the role of a buffer in conditions of acidosis and alkalosis. 5. Compare the roles of the respiratory system and the renal system in maintaining acid-base balance. 6. Describe the role of oxygen in maintaining acid-base balance. 7. Interpret whether the client's arterial blood gas values are normal, elevated, or low.	**Think-pair-share (3-5 min)** Complete TM 15-1 prior to class; compare answers. **Concept mapping (10-15 min)** Have learners draw an acid-base continuum. Place conditions that commonly cause acidosis on one end and place conditions that commonly cause alkalosis at the other end. Show the movement of hydrogen ions on the continuum. **Numbered heads together (5-10 min)** Ask learners any question that addresses any of the learning outcomes. **Send a problem (15-20 min)** Have learners write review questions on acid-base imbalances. Have learners write review questions on ABG findings in clients with acid-base imbalance.	**Transparency master** TM 15-1 Examples of disorders that are associated with acid-base imbalance **Internet resources** e-Kidneys.net: Acid-Base Balance http://www.e-kidneys.net/acidbase.html Musical Chemistry http://www.geocities.com/le_chatelier_uk/index.html **Community resources** Visit a support group for individuals with chronic respiratory problems—for example—chronic obstructive pulmonary disease (COPD) or emphysema. Analyze how members are coping. Ask them to relate their history of the disease. Have a respiratory therapist describe the collection of ABGs and their significance in a client's status.

Chapter 16: *Interventions for Clients with Acid-Base Imbalances*

Learning Outcomes	Learning Activities	Supplemental Resources
After studying this chapter, the student should be able to: 1. Identify clients at risk for acidosis. 2. Use laboratory data and clinical manifestations to determine the presence of acidosis. 3. Analyze arterial blood gases to determine whether acidosis is respiratory or metabolic in origin. 4. Analyze arterial blood gases to determine if respiratory acidosis is acute or chronic. 5. Prioritize nursing care for the client with acute acidosis. 6. Identify clients at risk for alkalosis. 7. Use laboratory data and clinical manifestations to determine the presence of alkalosis. 8. Analyze arterial blood gases to determine whether alkalosis is respiratory or metabolic in origin. 9. Prioritize nursing care for the client with alkalosis.	**Think-pair-share (3-5 min)** Complete TM 16-1 prior to class; compare answers. **Journaling (10-15 min)** Record experiences in caring for clients with acid-base imbalance, and fluid and electrolyte imbalances. **Concept mapping (15-20 min)** Have learners develop an interdisciplinary, comprehensive plan of care for a client with severe pulmonary emphysema who is experiencing respiratory acidosis; have them use a correlation mapping technique rather than a columnar care plan.	**Transparency master** TM 16-1 Arterial blood gas values for clients with acid-base imbalances **Internet resources** Virtual Hospital: Arterial Blood Gas Analysis http://www.vh.org/Providers/TeachingFiles/abg/Introduction.html **Community resources** Have a neonatal nurse from a tertiary care setting visit to discuss acid base problems encountered in neonates. Ask a nurse who works with clients who are ventilator dependent to speak about how acid-base problems are handled in this client population.

TM 11-1

LABORATORY FINDINGS IN THE CLIENT WITH DEHYDRATION

Laboratory Test	Change	Rationale
Blood urea nitrogen		
Serum creatinine		
Serum proteins		
Hematocrit/hemoglobin		
Urine-specific gravity		
Urine osmolarity		
Urine volume		

TM 12-1

COMPARISON OF FLUID DEFICIT AND FLUID OVERLOAD

	Fluid Deficit	**Fluid Overload**
Definition		
Types		
Clinical manifestations (includes laboratory findings)		
Collaborative management		

TM 15-1

EXAMPLES OF DISORDERS THAT ARE ASSOCIATED WITH ACID-BASE IMBALANCE

Acid-Base Imbalance	Examples of Common Disorders
Respiratory acidosis	
Metabolic acidosis	
Respiratory alkalosis	
Metabolic alkalosis	

TM 16-1

ARTERIAL BLOOD GAS VALUES FOR CLIENTS WITH ACID-BASE IMBALANCE

ABG Parameter	Respiratory Acidosis	Metabolic Acidosis	Respiratory Alkalosis	Metabolic Alkalosis
pH				
$PaCO_2$				
HCO_3				

Also indicate which values change during compensation.

UNIT 4 MANAGEMENT OF PERIOPERATIVE CLIENTS ■ Core Concepts Grid

Anatomy	Physiology	Pathophysiology	History	Physical Exam	Diagnostic Tests	Interventions	Pharmacology
			• **Age** • **Previous medical history** • **Tobacco** • **Usual medications** • **Previous surgeries** • **Complications of surgeries** • **Autologous blood donation** • **Support** • **Advance directions**	• **Vital signs** • **Breath sounds** • **Nutritional status** • **Exposure to infection** • **Cardiovascular system** • **Renal/urinary system** • **Neurologic system** • **Musculoskeletal system**	• **Routine urinalysis** • **Complete blood count** • **Blood urea nitrogen** • **Creatinine** • **Coagulation studies** • **Electrolyte studies** • **Electrocardiogram**	• **Preoperative** Surgical consent Pulmonary toilet Exercises to facilitate venous return Pain management Tubes Drains Dressings Intravenous fluids Skin preparation • **Intraoperative** Surgical team Nursing roles Holding area Positioning Anesthesia Complications Skin closures • **Postoperative** PACU assessment Return to unit Assessment Wound care Complications Infection Pulmonary embolism Deep vein thrombosis Paralytic ileus Dehiscence/ Evisceration Fluid management Tubes/drains Dressings Respiratory care Pain management Health teaching	• **Anesthetic agents** Intravenous Inhaled Spinal Local or regional • **Adjunct drugs** Hypnotics Opioids Blocking agents

Unit 4 (Chapters 17-19)

Management of Perioperative Clients

Learning Plan

Chapter 17: *Interventions for Preoperative Clients*

Learning Outcomes	Learning Activities	Supplemental Resources
After reading this chapter, the student should be able to: 1. Assume the role of client advocate. 2. Understand the legal implications and proper procedures for obtaining informed consent. 3. Prioritize teaching needs for the client preparing for surgery. 4. Describe client conditions or issues that need to be communicated to the surgical and postoperative teams.	**Think-pair-share (3-5 min)** What are the common reasons for surgery? Identify the common preoperative data that should be collected (include developmental considerations). Identify specific findings in the preoperative assessment that might lead to postoperative complications (include diagnostic findings). Can an emancipated minor sign his or her own surgical permit? Identify which clients are at risk for deep vein thrombosis. What should be done if it is discovered that a client did not sign the permit but has already received preoperative medication? **Pairs check (5 min)** Have pairs of learners identify the criteria for autologous blood donation, including the risks versus benefits of this type of blood donation. Have pairs of learners identify the factors involved in preoperative bowel preparation. Have pairs of learners teach each other the breathing and leg exercises and exercises used to prevent or reduce the severity of postoperative complications. **Journaling** Describe the anticipated emotional reactions of the preoperative client and his or her support persons (include developmental considerations). Describe the concerns the nurse might have for the preoperative client who takes antihypertensive or cardiac medications daily. How can the nurse best prepare the client for surgery that may be disfiguring?	**Internet resources** American Association of Nurse Anesthetists (AANA) http://www.aana.com/ American Society of PeriAnesthesia Nurses (ASPAN) http://www.aspan.org/ American Society of Plastic and Reconstructive Surgical Nurses (ASPSN) http://asprsn.inurse.com/ Association of Operating Room Nurses (AORN) http://www.aorn.org/

	Concept mapping Have learners map the elements of informed consent and identify data that would indicate that the conditions of informed consent have been met.	

Chapter 18: *Interventions for Intraoperative Clients*

Learning Outcomes	Learning Activities	Supplemental Resources
After reading this chapter, the student should be able to: 1. Discuss nursing interventions to reduce client and family anxiety. 2. Describe the roles and responsibilities of various intraoperative personnel. 3. Apply appropriate interventions to ensure the client's safety during an operative procedure. 4. Identify nursing responsibilities for management of clients receiving an anesthetic. 5. Recognize the clinical manifestations of malignant hyperthermia. 6. Apply appropriate interventions for the client experiencing malignant hyperthermia. 7. Discuss the potential adverse reactions and complications of specific anesthetic agents. 8. Assess clients for specific problems related to positioning during surgical procedures.	**Think-pair-share (5 min)** What factors influence the selection and dosage of anesthetics (include developmental considerations)? What assessment data in a client's history might indicate the potential for malignant hyperthermia? Identify the complications of intubation and the possible causes of the complication. Explain the techniques and indications for a medical aseptic versus a surgical aseptic scrub. **Pairs check (5 min)** Have pairs of learners prepare a chart outlining the advantages and disadvantages of the various types of inhalation anesthetics. Have pairs of learners describe various types of sutures. Each learner should be able to identify the purpose of a particular suture, typical tissue placement, and sizes. (Refer learner to illustration of sutures in chapter.) Have pairs of learners identify the uses, advantages, and possible complications of local or regional anesthesia. **Journaling and clinical component** Have learners observe or participate in surgery and identify the roles of the surgical team members. Discuss the ethical dilemmas that the nurse may encounter while acting on behalf of the client in regard to the Patient Self-Determination Act.	**Internet resources** American Association of Nurse Anesthetists (AANA) http://www.aana.com/ American Society of PeriAnesthesia Nurses (ASPAN) http://www.aspan.org/ American Society of Plastic Surgical Nurses (ASPSN) http://asprsn.inurse.com/ Association of Operating Room Nurses (AORN) http://www.aorn.org/ Discussion of the Patient Self-Determination Act http://www.springnet.com/ce/m710a.htm **Audiovisual** AORN: "Nursing: The Ultimate Adventure, Perioperative Edition"

Chapter 19: *Interventions for Postoperative Clients*

Learning Outcomes	Learning Activities	Supplemental Resources
After reading this chapter, the student should be able to: 1. Describe the ongoing head-to-toe assessment of the postoperative client. 2. Recognize wound complications in the postoperative period. 3. Prioritize common nursing interventions for the client recovering from surgery and anesthesia during the first 24 hours. 4. Prioritize nursing care for the client experiencing postoperative respiratory depression. 5. Discuss the criteria for determining readiness of the postoperative client to be discharged from the postanesthesia care unit. 6. Discuss the teaching priorities for postoperative clients.	**Think-pair-share (5 min)** What evidence would suggest that a client has experienced excessive blood loss during surgery? What impact does the mobility of today's family have on the client undergoing and recovering from surgery? Why is a client who is steroid dependent at risk for developing addisonian crisis? What impact might laser and laparoscopic surgery have on the postoperative period? Why might a client experience hypothermia in the postoperative period? What are the effects of malnutrition on wound healing? What are the possible etiologies of postoperative fever? **Pairs check (5 min)** Have pairs of learners calculate the number of calories in 1 L of 5% dextrose solution. (Use TM 19-1.) **Numbered heads together (10-15 min)** Form groups of two or three. Ask the groups to complete a comparison of opioid and nonopioid drugs used for pain control prior to coming to class. In class, after numbering the groups, ask even numbered groups to list the advantages and disadvantages of opioid drugs and odd numbered groups to list the advantages and disadvantages of nonopioid drugs. (Use TM 19-2.) Form groups of two or three, as groups are available, and have each group complete one component of Chart 19-3. Allow each group to present its findings so that each learner has a completed chart. **Structured controversy (10-15 min)** The client who is HIV positive should not have surgery. The health care worker who is HIV positive should be allowed to be a member of the surgical team.	**Transparency masters** TM 19-1 Level of 5% Dextrose Solution TM 19-2 Pain Drug Comparison Worksheet 19-3 **Internet resources** American Association of Nurse Anesthetists (AANA) http://www.aana.com/ American Society of PeriAnesthesia Nurses (ASPAN) http://www.aspan.org/ American Society of Plastic and Reconstructive Surgical Nurses (ASPRSN) http://asprsn.inurse.com/ Association of Operating Room Nurses (AORN) http://www.aorn.org/ Discussion of the Patient Self-Determination Act http://www.springnet.com/ce/m710a.htm

	Journaling and clinical component How has the increasing use of ambulatory surgery changed the role of the perioperative nurse? **Concept mapping** Ask learners to map the events that occur in the postoperative period linking the common assessments with the events they identify.	

TM 19-1

5% Dextrose/Water

1000 mL

Sterile Nonpyrogenic

Single-Dose Container

Each 100 mL contains:
5g Dextrose Hydrous USP pH 4.0 (3.2 to 6.5)
Osmolarity 252 mOsmo/L (calc)

Additives may be incompatible. When introducing additives, use aseptic technique. Mix thoroughly. Do not store.

Dosage: Intravenously as directed by a physician. See directions.

Cautions: Inspect inner bag, which maintains product sterility. Discard if leaks are found. Must not be used in series connections. Do not administer simultaneously with blood. Do not use unless solution is clear. Federal law prohibits dispensing without prescription. Store unit in moistureproof barrier at room temperature until ready to use. Avoid excessive heat. See package insert or consult pharmacist for further information.

TM 19-2

PAIN DRUG COMPARISON: OPIOID AND NONOPIOID DRUGS USED FOR PERIOPERATIVE PAIN CONTROL

Drug	Class	Usual Dose/Route	Side/Adverse Effects	Nursing Implications
Morphine SO_4				
Meperidine HCl (Demerol)				
Codeine				
Acetaminophen (Tylenol)				
Ibuprofen (Motrin) (or other NSAID)				
Hydroxyzine HCl (Vistaril)				
Fentanyl (Sublimaze)				

TM 19-3

POSTOPERATIVE ASSESSMENT TOOL

For each body system, include what the assessment parameters are, what the possible abnormalities are, and what the findings might indicate.

System	Findings	Indications
Respiratory		
Cardiovascular		
Fluids/Hydration		
Neurologic		
Gastrointestinal		
Integument (include dressings/drains)		

CHAPTER 17

Case Study for the Preoperative Client

A 49-year-old client with a history of hypertension is scheduled for a total hysterectomy. Her hypertension is controlled by Avapro. She has a history of excessive vaginal bleeding. Her latest hemoglobin and hematocrit levels were 9 g/dL and 26%, respectively. The client tells you that she has a great fear of a blood transfusion. She has complaints of tiredness and easy fatigue. You are the preadmission surgical nurse.

Questions

1. What information could you relay to the client about autologous blood transfusions?

2. Name three factors the preadmission surgical nurse should evaluate in regard to this client.

3. What would you teach the client about the immediate postoperative period regarding chest physiotherapy and vaginal discharge?

CHAPTER 18

Case Study for the Intraoperative Client

You are an OR nurse having lunch in the hospital cafeteria with one of your friends who works in the open-heart surgery unit. He tells you that, "Boy, we seem to get a lot of clients out of the OR with skin breakdown on the back of their heads." Upon further discussion, he tells you that most often the breakdown is black eschar.

Questions

1. Is it possible that these clients developed the skin breakdown while in the operating suite? Why or why not?

2. What should you do with the information your friend passed on to you and why?

3. How could these situations have been prevented?

CHAPTER 19

Case Study for the Postoperative Client

You are a nurse working on a medical-surgical unit, and midway through your shift you are notified that your postoperative client was just placed in his room. You had not received any notice that you were receiving any client in that room, nor did you get any report.

Questions

1. What do you do first?

2. What do you say to the client?

3. What action should you take regarding not being notified of the admission and not receiving a report?

UNIT 5 PROBLEMS OF PROTECTION ■ Core Concepts Grid

Anatomy	Physiology	Pathophysiology	History	Physical Exam	Diagnostic Tests	Interventions	Pharmacology
• **Lymph system** • **Mononuclear—phagocyte system** • **Cells** B-lymphocytes T-lymphocytes • **Antigens**	• **Phagocytosis** • **Specificity** • **Memory** • **Self-recognition** • **Human leukocyte antigen (HLA)** • **Inflammatory response** • **Immune response** Antibody-mediated Cell-mediated • **Types of immunity** Natural Acquired Active Passive	• **Hypersensitivity response** • **Autoimmune response** • **Immunodeficiency** • **Metastasis** • **Neoplasm** • **Inflammation** • **Infection** • **Transplant reaction** • **Tissue degeneration**	• **Past history of infections, allergies, malignancies, autoimmune disease** • **Immunization record** • **Family history** • **Social history** Occupation Nutrition	• **Liver size and location** • **Spleen** • **Thymus** • **Lymphatic system** Nodes • **Fever** • **Skin rashes** • **Urticaria** • **Itching** • **Fatigue** • **Malaise** • **Infection** • **Respiratory distress** • **Weight loss** • **Joint assessment** • **Cardiovascular system** • **Renal system**	• **Complete blood count** • **Carcinoembryonic antigen (CEA)** • **C-reactive protein** • **Immunoglobins IgA, IgG, IgM, IgD, IgE** • **Rheumatoid factor** • **Antinuclear antibody titer** • **Enzyme-linked immunosorbent assay (ELISA)** • **Western blot** • **Skin tests** • **Tumor staging**	• **Education** Avoidance of infection Avoidance of trigger substances • **Rest** • **Nutrition** • **Stress management** • **Lifestyle alterations** • **Radiation** • **Bone marrow transplantation** • **Therapeutic exercise** • **Energy conservation** • **Joint protection** • **Skin protection from the sun** • **Joint replacement** Total hip Total knee • **Abduction pillow** • **Continuous passive motion (CPM) machine** • **Postoperative complications** Infection Thromboembolitic complications Dislocation	• **Histamine blockers** • **Corticosteroids** • **Hyposensitization** • **Immunosuppressants** • **Chemotherapeutic agents** • **Biologic response modifiers (BRMs)** • **Antibiotics** • **Nonsteroidal anti-inflammatory drugs** • **Opioids**

Unit 5 (Chapters 20-26)

Problems of Protection: Management of Clients with Problems of the Immune System

Learning Plan

Chapter 20: *Concepts of Inflammation and the Immune Response*

Learning Outcomes	Learning Activities	Supplemental Resources
After reading this chapter, the student should be able to: 1. Describe the concept of self-tolerance. 2. Explain the difference between inflammation and infection. 3. Compare and contrast the cells, purposes, and features of inflammation and immunity. 4. Describe the basis for the five cardinal manifestations of inflammation. 5. Interpret a white blood cell count with differential to indicate no immune problems, an acute bacterial infection, a chronic bacterial infection, or an allergic reaction. 6. Explain how complement activation and fixation assists in protection from infection. 7. Compare the cells, function, and protective actions of antibody-mediated immunity and cell-mediated immunity. 8. Compare and contrast the types of antibody-mediated immunities.	**Think-pair-share (5 min)** Identify and discuss the stages of the inflammatory response. Identify the function of neutrophils, macrophages, basophils, and eosinophils. Differentiate between acute rejection and chronic rejection according to the time frame involved, specific findings, and outcomes. Differentiate among innate-native immunity, acquired immunity, and cell-mediated immunity. Identify the symptoms of rejection of transplanted organs. State the reasons why kidney and liver transplant failure is high because of rejection. Describe treatment of transplant rejection. Discuss the effects that vitamin and mineral supplements may have on improving the immune function in the older adult. **Concept mapping (15 min)** Ask learners to draw a map of the organization of the immune system. Ask learners to draw a map of the physiology of inflammation that includes the five cardinal physical manifestations of inflammation: warmth, redness, swelling, pain, and decreased function. Ask learners to draw a map of the seven steps of antibody production.	**Internet resources** Graft vs. Host Disease http://www.med.jhu.edu/cancerctr/hematol/gvh.htm National Institute of Allergy and Infectious Diseases http://www.niaid.nih.gov/final/immds/immds.htm **Community resources** State Health Department Annual AIDS Surveillance Reports Centers for Disease Control Morbidity and Mortality Weekly Report (MMWR) List of HIV/AIDS Materials. CAC National AIDS Clearinghouse (1-800-458-5231) Regional AIDS Education and Training Centers e.g., Mountain-Plains Regional AIDS Education and Training Center Southeast AIDS Education and Training Center

	Pairs share (15 min) Using the supposition that the pairs are a nurse and a family member of a client receiving a transplant, have one member of the team role play the nurse and teach the other member the signs and symptoms of hyperacute rejection. Switch roles and provide teaching about the signs and symptoms of acute rejection. Allow each scenario family member participant to ask questions of the "nurse." **Journaling** Ask learners to describe the nurse's role in dealing with the client who has had to have a rejected organ removed.	

Chapter 21: *Interventions for Clients with Connective Tissue Disease*

Learning Outcomes	Learning Activities	Supplemental Resources
After reading this chapter, the student should be able to: 1. Compare and contrast the pathophysiology and clinical manifestations of degenerative joint disease (DJD) and rheumatoid disease (RA). 2. Discuss the priority collaborative interventions for clients with DJD and RA. 3. Determine common nursing diagnoses for postoperative clients having total joint replacement. 4. Evaluate the expected outcomes for clients' total joint replacement surgery. 5. Interpret laboratory findings for clients with rheumatoid disease. 6. Discuss the differences between discoid lupus erythematosus and systemic lupus erythematosus.	**Think-pair-share (5 min)** Identify changes seen with a dislocated hip prosthesis. Compare the symptoms with those of a fractured hip. Discuss the rationale for and methods of weight reduction as a treatment for arthritis. Describe diet therapy variations in the various connective tissue disorders. In any client, why is infection of the bone so serious? Include in your discussion the length of treatment. What laboratory tests might best differentiate between degenerative joint disease and rheumatoid arthritis? (Use Worksheet 21-1.) Explain why plasmapheresis is used to remove antibodies in clients with SLE. Discuss methods and alternate positions for sexual intercourse that might be used by clients and their partners after hip or knee replacement. How does connective tissue disease affect the future of clients across the age continuum?	**Transparency masters** TM 21-1 Comparison of Rheumatoid Arthritis and Degenerative Joint Disease **Internet resources** Arthritis Foundation http://www.arthritis.org/ Arthritis Links http://arthritis.miningco.com/msub29.htm http://www.orthop.washington.edu/ Arthritis National Research Foundation http://www.curearthritis.org/ John Hopkins Arthritis Center http://www.hopkins-arthritis.som.jhmi.edu/

<table>
<tr>
<td>7. Identify client education needs for clients with arthritis.
8. Differentiate between discoid lupus erythematosus and systemic lupus erythematosus.
9. Describe the priority nursing interventions for clients who have progressive systemic sclerosis.
10. Identify the pathophysiology and etiology of gout.
11. Explain the differences among polymyositis, systemic necrotizing vasculitis, polymyalgia rheumatica, ankylosing spondylitis, Reiter's syndrome, and Sjögren's syndrome.
12. Describe interventions that clients can use to prevent Lyme disease.
13. Identify the primary concern in care for clients with Marfan syndrome.
14. Describe the common clinical manifestations of fibromyalgia.</td>
<td>Pairs share (15 min)
Using the supposition that the pairs are a nurse and a family member of a client with DJD, have one member of the team role play the nurse and teach the other member the signs and symptoms of DJD. Switch roles and provide teaching about the signs and symptoms of RA. Allow each scenario family member participant to ask questions of the "nurse."
Ask a physical therapist to demonstrate the continuous passive motion (CPM) machine. Have one learner role play as the client and one learner discuss the care and teaching of the clients with this intervention. Have them reverse roles. Describe the criteria for increasing the degree of flexion.
Have learners develop a teaching plan for crutch walking gaits (the three-point is the most common).

Numbered heads together (5-7 min)
Ask even-numbered learners to identify the common pharmacological management of degenerative joint disease. Have odd-numbered learners identify the common pharmacological management of rheumatoid arthritis.

Campus lab/Clinical component (10-15 min)
Set up an orthopedic bed with various types of traction, slings, and splints for learners to examine. Place learners in various forms of skin traction, use of adduction pillow, etc.
Examine an x-ray of a client with arthritis and a normal x-ray of the same joint. (The joint with arthritis has a cloudy area in the joint space, whereas the normal joint has a crisp separation.)
Have pairs of learners practice applying antiembolism stockings and sequential compression devices to one another in the clinical laboratory setting.</td>
<td>Arthritis Research Institute of America (ARIS)
http://www.preventarthritis.org/

Lupus Foundation of America
http://www.lupus.org/lupus/

Sjogren's syndrome
http://www.sjogrens.com/

Gout
http://www.arthritis.org/answers/diseasecenter/gout.asp

American Lyme Disease Foundation
http://www.aldf.com/</td>
</tr>
</table>

	Concept mapping (15 min) Ask learners to develop a concept map by systems of the many manifestations of systemic lupus erythematosus. **Journaling** Some health care workers have described a "rheumatoid personality" as a very demanding, hostile person. Explore how this personality may be attributed to the continuous pain and deformity experienced by the client. **Structured controversy** What ethical issues occur when many people wait until they are over 65 years old to have a joint replacement and are eligible for Medicare in the United States? Does this place an unnecessary burden on society for the cost? Do these implications change in countries with universal health coverage? Should joint replacement surgery be performed on obese clients who have joint damage and joint pain due to the excess weight?	

Chapter 22: *Interventions for Clients with HIV and Other Immunodeficiencies*

Learning Outcomes	Learning Activities	Supplemental Resources
After reading this chapter, the student should be able to: 1. Compare and contrast primary versus secondary immunodeficiencies for causes and onset of problems. 2. Explain the differences in nursing care required for a client with a pathogenic infection versus a client with an opportunistic infection. 3. Distinguish between the conditions of human immunodeficiency virus (HIV) infection and acquired immunodeficiency syndrome (AIDS) for clinical manifestations and risks for complications.	**Think-pair-share (5 min)** What data are pertinent in the history and physical examination of a client with AIDS? Describe the skin lesions seen with Kaposi's sarcoma. What are the central and peripheral nervous system effects of AIDS? How might a nurse collect a complete history and perform a physical examination on a client with AIDS? What is the role of CD4 (an antigen on the surface of helper T cells)? What various opportunistic infections associated with HIV infection and AIDS may have an impact on nutrition?	**Internet resources** National Center for HIV, STD, and TB Prevention. Divisions of HIV/AIDS Prevention http://www.cdc.gov/hiv/dhap.htm HIV/AIDS Treatment Information Service (ATIS) http://www.hivatis.org/ AIDS Research Information Center http://www.critpath.org/aric/ HIV/AIDS Resources, Center for Disease Control http://www.cdcnpin.org/hiv/

4. Describe the ways in which HIV is transmitted. 5. Identify techniques to reduce the risk for infection in an immunocompromised client. 6. Develop a teaching plan for condom use among sexually active non–English speaking adults. 7. Prioritize care for the client with AIDS who has impaired gas exchange. 8. Identify teaching priorities for the HIV-positive client receiving highly active antiretroviral therapy. 9. Plan a week of meals for the client who has protein-calorie malnutrition. 10. Describe the nursing actions and responsibilities for administration of IV immunoglobulin.	What laboratory values and the data they provide can better indicate immunocompetence? What are some specific sites of action of AIDS drugs? Why do opportunistic infections sometimes follow long-term antibiotic therapy? What are the complications of AIDS that require surgery, and what are the necessary precautions for these procedures? What are the needs for care of a client with AIDS at home? **Campus lab/Clinical component (10-15 min)** Assess whether your clients are prone to opportunistic infections. **Concept mapping (15 min)** Ask learners to develop a concept of opportunistic infections. **Structured controversy (10-15 min)** An HIV-positive individual or a person with AIDS should be allowed to attend nursing school anonymously. Discuss the impact of AIDS on the medical system and the legal and ethical implications for children born to AIDS-infected mothers. AIDS clients should not be eligible for TPN and organ transplants. Private insurance companies should be allowed to raise rates for people who are at high risk of acquiring AIDS. A person with AIDS who purposefully contaminates another person should be charged with murder. **Campus lab/Clinical component (10-15 min)** Demonstrate the procedure for cleanup of a blood spill. **Journaling** What are some of the most difficult personal feelings with which a nurse must deal in caring for clients with AIDS?	Agency for Health Care Research and Quality http://www.ahrq.gov/

Chapter 23: *Interventions for Clients with Immune Function Excess: Hypersensitivity (Allergy) and Autoimmunity*

Learning Outcomes	Learning Activities	Supplemental Resources
After reading this chapter, the student should be able to: 1. Compare and contrast the bases for and manifestations of allergy and autoimmunity. 2. Discuss the nursing responsibility for a client experiencing anaphylaxis. 3. Describe allergy testing techniques. 4. List the defining characteristics of type I, type II, type III, type IV, and type V hypersensitivity reactions. 5. Explain the differences in mechanisms of action between antihistamines and mast cell stabilizers.	**Think-pair-share (5 min)** What is the rationale for and cellular action of antihistamines, corticosteroids, and epinephrine given for allergic reactions? What are the roles of IgM, IgA, IgG, and IgE in disease? What is known about a cure for the common cold? What is the rationale for the discontinuation of systemic corticosteroids or antihistamines prior to allergy testing? What is the difference between type I, type II, type III, type IV, and type IV reactions? **Pairs check** Ask learners to analyze their client's WBC levels and explain why certain values are elevated (for example, allergies with eosinophils and infection with neutrophils). **Concept mapping (15 min)** Ask learners to map the concept of the immune system as a surveillance mechanism. Ask learners to map the process of desensitization therapy. Ask learners to map the relationship between anaphylaxis and therapeutic management of symptoms. **Numbered heads together (15 min)** Ask learners to draw an algorithm to differentiate the body's reaction to injection with a sterile nail versus a rusty nail. Ask learners to examine the WBC counts of a client with a viral infection and one with a bacterial infection. Compare and contrast the values.	**Internet resources** The American Academy of Allergy, Asthma and Immunology http://www.aaaai.org/ Allergy, Asthma & Immunology Online http://www.allergy.mcg.edu/ **Community resources** Have learners spend the morning in a local allergist office. What precautions are taken should a client experience an allergic response? Have learners evaluate the difference between skin testing and other methods of allergy testing.

Chapter 24: *Altered Cell Growth and Cancer Development*

Learning Outcomes	Learning Activities	Supplemental Resources
After reading this chapter, the student should be able to: 1. Explain why cause of cancer can be hard to establish. 2. Compare and contrast the characteristics of benign and malignant tumors. 3. List three cancer types associated with exposure to tobacco. 4. Identify cancer types for which primary prevention is possible. 5. Compare and contrast the cancer development processes of initiation and promotion. 6. Describe the TNM system for cancer staging. 7. Explain the differences between a "low-grade" cancer and a "high-grade" cancer. 8. Discuss the role of oncogenes and suppressor genes in cancer development. 9. Identify four common sites of distant metastasis for cancer. 10. Discuss the role of immunity in protection against cancer. 11. Identify which cancer types arise from connective tissues and which types arise from glandular tissues. 12. Describe how genetic predisposition can increase a person's risk for cancer development. 13. Identify behaviors that reduce the risk for cancer development and cancer death.	**Think-pair-share (5 min)** Compare and contrast the growth cycles in benign versus malignant tumors. How is a tumor graded, and how is cancer disease staged? What is the role of bone marrow transplant in the treatment of cancers? Identify the steps of metastasis. What extrinsic factors are involved in cancer development? What intrinsic factors are involved in cancer development? **Numbered heads together (15 min)** Have learners draw a benign tumor and a malignant tumor. Then ask them to draw a metastatic tumor and look for similarities in the cell type from the parent tumor to the metastatic site. **Concept mapping** Have learners, beginning with a central cell, draw a map distinguishing the biology of growth of a normal cell on one side from the biology of growth of an abnormal cell from the other side. **Structured controversy** Explore the process of metastasis and characteristics of the metastatic cell being like the parent cell. **Campus lab/Clinical component** Review the charts of clients with cancer. With the TNM system, what stage is each client's cancer? Share this information with your clinical group.	**Internet resources** The American Cancer Society http://www.cancer.org/ The American Association for Cancer Research http://www.aacr.org/ Memorial Sloan-Kettering Cancer Center http://www.mskcc.org/

Chapter 25: *Interventions for Clients with Cancer*

Learning Outcomes	Learning Activities	Supplemental Resources
After reading this chapter, the student should be able to: 1. Identify the goals of cancer therapy. 2. Differentiate between cancer surgery for cure and cancer surgery for palliation. 3. Discuss how the nursing care needs for the client undergoing surgery compare with those for the client undergoing any other type of surgery. 4. Compare and contrast the purposes and side effects of radiation therapy and chemotherapy for cancer. 5. Prioritize nursing care for the client with radiation-induced skin problems. 6. Prioritize education needs for the client receiving external beam radiation. 7. Compare the personnel safety issues for working with clients receiving teletherapy radiation versus those receiving brachytherapy radiation. 8. Identify nursing interventions to promote safety for the client experiencing chemotherapy-induced anemia or thrombocytopenia. 9. Prioritize nursing care for the client with chemotherapy-induced neutropenia. 10. Prioritize nursing care for the client with mucositis. 11. Explain the rationale for hormonal manipulation therapy. 12. Discuss the uses of biologic response modifiers as supportive therapy in the treatment of cancer. 13. Identify clients at risk for oncologic emergencies.	**Think-pair-share (5 min)** Describe the assessment of the client with cancer. Compare the incidence of cancer in tribal people, who eat fresh fruits and vegetables, roots, and grasses, with the higher incidence in sedentary North Americans, who eat more red meat. What changes occur in lung tissue after a client stops smoking cigarettes? Discuss the current projections of cancer occurrence from the American Cancer Society for expected incidence and mortality by age, gender, and site. What extrinsic factors in the diet may increase the risk of cancer? Identify various modalities of nutritional therapy for the client with cancer. Consider interventions for nausea, vomiting, diarrhea, and stomatitis. Why do cancer cells and normal highly mitotic cells die during radiation and chemotherapy? Why is hypercalcemia indicative of bone cancer? **Pairs check (15 min)** Have the learners demonstrate oral mucosa assessment techniques. Describe objective means to assess the oral mucosa and the continuing need for oral care in the client with drug-induced stomatitis. **Concept mapping (15 min)** Ask learners to complete the cell-cycle drug comparison table prior to class. Ask even-numbered learners to state the advantages of cell-cycle–specific agents and disadvantages of cell-cycle–nonspecific agents. Ask odd-numbered learners to state the advantages of cell-cycle–nonspecific agents and disadvantages of cell-cycle–specific agents. Ask each group to identify cancer cell characteristics that could best be treated with a cell-cycle–specific agent or cell-cycle–nonspecific agent. (Use TM 25-1.) Ask learners to map the mechanism of action of radiation therapy.	**Transparency masters** TM 25-1 Comparison of cell-cycle–specific agents and cell-cycle–nonspecific agents **Internet resources** The American Cancer Society http://www.cancer.org/ American Institute for Cancer Research http://www.aicr.org/ American Society of Clinical Oncology http://www.asco.org/ Harvard Center for Cancer Prevention http://www.yourcancerrisk.harvard.edu/ oncology.com http://www.oncology.com/ National Cancer Institute http://www.nci.nih.gov/

	Journaling Have learners explore their personal risks for cancer. What is the home care preparation for the client with cancer? Explore the fact that cancer is a parasite to its host and relate this to development of emaciation in the client. Discuss the implications for discovery of the genes that indicate a person is a carrier for or has increased susceptibility to various types of cancer. What are the financial considerations? What are the emotional considerations? What are the implications for health care insurance eligibility if a person is a known carrier of the gene? Discuss the nurse's role in talking to clients who have chosen to obtain illegal or unproven treatment for cancer, such as megavitamins. **Campus lab/Clinical component (10-15 min)** Identify methods to protect the staff from the toxic effects of the chemotherapeutic agents and implantable radium. Manage the care of clients receiving chemotherapeutic agents. **Structured controversy (10-15 min)** Carcinogenic items should not be allowed on the open market. Discuss the impact on the economy if tobacco, food dyes, and pollutants were illegal. Could they be stopped all together? Cancer should not be treated if the prognosis is poor.	

Chapter 26: *Interventions for Clients with Infection*

Learning Outcomes	Learning Activities	Supplemental Resources
After reading this chapter, the student should be able to: 1. Explain the chain of infection. 2. Describe the principles of infection control in inpatient and community-based setting. 3. Discuss the risk of gloves and other products made with latex. 4. Interpret the four types of transmission-based precautions. 5. Identify the major complications of infection. 6. Describe the common clinical manifestations of infection for which the nurse should assess. 7. Interpret laboratory test findings related to infections and infectious diseases. 8. Evaluate nursing interventions for fever management.	**Think-pair-share (5 min)** Describe the single most important intervention to interrupt the chain of infection. What factors in the skin facilitate a defense against infection? What is the financial impact of nosocomial infections? Why are nosocomial infections more difficult to treat? Why might recent animal contact lead the nurse to suspect an increased risk for infection? Why must culture and sensitivity testing be performed before the initiation of antibiotic therapy? **Pairs check (15 min)** Have the learners describe the purpose of culture and sensitivity testing, including the nurse's role in collection of specimens. **Concept mapping (15 min)** Ask learners to map the chain of infection including examples of each link in the chain. **Campus lab/Clinical component (10-15 min)** Examine the gloves used by health care workers at your facility. Are they latex free, or are latex-free gloves an option? Examine the setups for each type of isolation precautions.	**Internet resources** The Chain of Infection http://web54.sd54.k12.il.us/schools/addams/dmoore/chain_site.htm Center for Clinical Epidemiology http://www.apic.org/cce/ Center for Disease Control http://www.cdc.gov/ **Community resources** Have groups of learners develop a teaching demonstration of appropriate handwashing techniques. Have them visit local grade schools and teach students the technique.

TM 21-1

COMPARISON OF RHEUMATOID ARTHRITIS AND DEGENERATIVE JOINT DISEASE

Disease	**Etiology**	**Pathogenesis**	**Common Lab Tests**	**Treatments**
Rheumatoid arthritis (RA)				
Degenerative joint disease (DJD)				

TM 25-1

COMPARISON OF CELL-CYCLE–SPECIFIC AND CELL-CYCLE–NONSPECIFIC AGENTS

Drug	Cell-Cycle–Specific (CCS)/Cell-Cycle–Nonspecific (CCNS)	Class	Action
Methotrexate (Mexate) 5 Fluorouracil (5-FU)			
Bleomycin (Blenoxane) Mithramycin (Mithracin)			
Cyclophosphamide (Cytoxan) Cisplatin (Platinol)			
Vincristine (Oncovin) Paclitaxel (Taxol)			
Procarbazine (Matulane) L-Asparaginase (Elspar)			

CHAPTER 21

Case Study for the Client with Systemic Lupus Erythematosus

A 32-year-old white female client with complaints of a facial rash comes to the physician's office where you are a nurse. On further questioning, you find that she has been more fatigued than usual and has an achy left ankle. Her infant son is 4 months old, and she has just stopped bleeding from her traumatic vaginal delivery (the baby weighed 10 pounds and she was in labor for 18 hours.)

Questions

1. When taking a complete history, what other questions should you ask the client at this time?

2. If she has systemic lupus erythematosus (SLE), what other clinical manifestations might she have?

3. What risk factors does she have for SLE?

4. What laboratory tests will the physician most likely order?

CHAPTER 22

Case Study for the Client with AIDS

A 32-year-old woman is one of your home-care clients with AIDS. Her medication orders include TMP, 160 mg BID; SMX, 800 mg BID; ketoconazole, 200 mg QD; didanosine, 200 mg BID. Today, she complains that she is short of breath and has sharp pains in her chest. She appears anxious. During the respiratory assessment, you find that she is dyspneic and tachypneic at rest, with a respiratory rate of 30/min. On auscultation, you hear crackles in her right lower lobe.

Questions

1. When taking the client's history, what important questions should you ask?

2. What physical assessment techniques should you perform?

3. Given the respiratory findings, what should you do first?

PROBLEMS OF OXYGENATION: RESPIRATORY TRACT ■ Core Concepts Grid

Anatomy	Physiology	Pathophysiology	History	Physical Exam	Diagnostic Tests	Interventions	Pharmacology
• **Upper respiratory tract** • **Lower respiratory tract** • **Alveolar level** • **Thoracic structure**	• **Ventilation** • **Thoracic pressure**	• **Obstruction** • **Inflammation** • **Trauma** • **Hypoxia** • **Infection** • **Fibrosis** • **Tumor** • **Respiratory failure**	• **Risk factors** Smoking Age Occupation Previous health Socioeconomic status • **Cardinal symptoms** Fatigue Cough Sputum Chest pain • **Growth and development**	• **Respiratory rate, rhythm, depth** • **Breath sounds** • **Dyspnea** • **Cyanosis/pallor** • **Restlessness** • **Irritability** • **Confusion** • **Hoarseness** • **Dysrhythmias**	• **Chest x-ray** • **Arterial blood gas (ABG)** • **Pulse oximetry** • **Lung volumes** • **Sputum cultures** • **Acid-fast bacillus** • **Bronchoscopy** • **Thoracentesis** • **Complete blood count** • **V/Q lung scan**	• **Positioning** • **Oxygen** • **Incentive spirometry** • **Chest physiotherapy** • **Postural drainage** • **Breathing techniques** • **Intubation** Endotracheal Tracheotomy Tracheostomy • **Suction** • **Chest tubes** • **Mechanical ventilation** • **Lung transplantation** • **Health teaching**	• **Antitussives** • **Anti-infectives** Antibiotics Antituberculars • **Bronchodilators** • **Mucolytics** • **Anti-inflammatory drugs** • **Corticosteroids** • **Chemotherapeutic agents** • **Anticoagulants**

Unit 6 (Chapters 27-32)

Problems of Oxygenation: Management of Clients with Problems of the Respiratory Tract

Learning Plan

Chapter 27: *Assessment of the Respiratory System*

Learning Outcomes	Learning Activities	Supplemental Resources
After reading this chapter, the student should be able to: 1. Compare and contrast the structure and functions of the upper airways to those of the lower airways. 2. Distinguish between normal and abnormal (adventitious) breath sounds. 3. Describe the respiratory changes associated with aging. 4. Calculate the pack-year smoking history for the client who smokes or who has ever smoked cigarettes. 5. Demonstrate proper technique when using observation and auscultation to assess the respiratory system. 6. Demonstrate proper technique when using palpation and percussion to assess the respiratory system. 7. Interpret arterial blood gas values to assess the client's respiratory status. 8. Prioritize education needs for the client undergoing pulmonary function tests. 9. Prioritize nursing care for the client after bronchosopy or open lung biopsy.	**Concept mapping** Have learners map the nursing care involved for the client undergoing thoracentesis compared with the client undergoing lung biopsy. **Think-pair-share (5-10 min)** What does the pulse oximeter measure? How does the information from an arterial blood gas report differ from the information from a pulse oximeter? Explain the mechanism that controls the respiratory rate in the healthy individual. Give groups of learners worksheets with several arterial blood gas values. Ask them to identify the acid-base state, whether metabolic or respiratory, acidosis or alkalosis and state the presence of any compensation. Each group should take turns interpreting a blood gas report. **Campus lab/Clinical component (10-15 min)** In a learning lab setting, have learners perform inspection, palpation, auscultation, and percussion of the thorax on a partner. Bring a pulse oximeter to class. Demonstrate how it is applied and how to operate the machine. Calculate pack years of smoking for someone who has smoked two packs a day for 12 years.	**Internet resources** Lung function fundamentals http://www.anaesthetist.com/icu/organs/lung/lungfx.htm Structure and Function of the Lung http://edcenter.med.cornell.edu/CUMC_PathNotes/Respiratory/Respiratory.html Interpretation of Pulmonary Function Tests: Spirometry http://www.vh.org/Providers/Simulations/Spirometry/SpirometryHome.html An Overview of Pulmonary Function Tests http://www.slowhand.net/drpr/pfts.htm **Community resources** Have groups of learners investigate community smoking cessation programs for issues such as cost to the participant, convenience of program hours, and program success. Have groups of learners visit local chapter of the American Lung Association or the American Cancer Association and obtain literature and programs on smoking cessation. Have all nursing students present and promote the Great American Smokeout day on their campus.

Chapter 28: *Interventions for Clients with Oxygen or Tracheostomy*

Learning Outcomes	Learning Activities	Supplemental Resources
After reading this chapter, the student should be able to: 1. Compare and contrast the uses and nursing care issues of oxygen delivery by mask with oxygen delivery by nasal cannula. 2. Explain the problems associated with oxygen therapy for those clients whose respiratory efforts are controlled by the hypoxic drive. 3. Analyze changes in clinical manifestations to determine the effectiveness of therapy for the client receiving oxygen. 4. Use laboratory data and clinical manifestations to determine the presence of hypoxemia or hypercarbia. 5. Prioritize nursing care for the client with a new trachesotomy. 6. Identify techniques to minimize the risk for aspiration when helping the client with a trachesotomy.	**Concept mapping** Assign learners to groups of four and ask them to map oxygenation. Learners should be directed to include as many ideas as they can generate about oxygenation in 5 minutes. At the end of 5 minutes, each group should give its map to a different group and continue the process. At the end of 5 more minutes, have one group present, then have each group add any additional information. **Think-pair-share (5 min)** Which requires more energy, inhalation or exhalation? Explain the mechanism that controls respiration in the healthy individual. When and why does the hypoxic drive occur? Argue the statement that although oxygen therapy is a serious concern, untreated or inadequately treated hypoxemia is a greater threat to life. What is the purpose of humidification of oxygen? What are the priority nursing interventions in tracheostomy tube dislodgment or decannulation? What are the nursing interventions for preventing hypoxia during suctioning for a client undergoing a tracheostomy? **Numbered heads together (10-15 min)** Ask learners to complete a worksheet listing the advantages and disadvantages of various oxygen delivery systems (Worksheet 28-1). Ask the even-numbered learners in a group to identify the client advantages of the various types of oxygen delivery equipment. Ask the odd-numbered learners to identify the client disadvantages for the various types of oxygen delivery equipment. Develop an algorithm for selecting the appropriate oxygen delivery system.	**Internet resources** Oxygen Delivery Systems http://www.fi.edu/biosci/systems/respiration.html Oxygen Concentration and Delivery to Tissues http://www.therox.com/o2concentration.htm **Community resources** Have groups of learners determine how to obtain oxygen delivery systems at home. Have a second group solve this dilemma. Sally, a 65-year-old with a history of emphysema, has just started receiving oxygen full-time. She has been lap swimming on a daily basis and wants to continue this practice. She asks how she can do this and still use her oxygen. What is available to her?

	Campus lab/Clinical component (10-15 min) Differentiate between the various types of tracheostomy tubes. Demonstrate the appropriate technique for the care and cleaning of a tracheostomy. **Journaling** What can the nurse do to support the client with a tracheostomy who is dealing with body image disturbances?	

Chapter 29: ***Interventions for Clients with Noninfectious Upper Respiratory Problems***

Learning Outcomes	Learning Activities	Supplemental Resources
After reading this chapter, the student should be able to: 1. Compare the clinical manifestations and care needs of a client with an anterior nosebleed with those of a client with a posterior nosebleed. 2. Prioritize the nursing care needs of a client with facial trauma. 3. Identify the potential complications of sleep apnea. 4. Develop a plan of communication for a client who has a disruption of speech and cannot read. 5. Use clinical manifestations and laboratory data to determine airway adequacy in a client with laryngeal or neck injury. 6. Identify the risk factors that predispose a client to the development of head and neck cancer.	**Think-pair-share (3-5 min)** Identify and place in priority the nursing interventions anticipated following rhinoplasty. What are the factors that contribute to sleep apnea? Identify the pathophysiology behind five of the causes of upper airway obstruction. Discuss the advantages and disadvantages of the interventions for upper airway obstruction. What are the anticipated complications of a head and neck resection? Develop a plan to meet the early and ongoing nutritional needs of the client after laryngectomy. **Concept mapping** Pair learners and have them role play taking a history from a client with an assigned respiratory problem. Direct learners to reverse roles, select a different respiratory problem, and again role play taking a history. Pair learners and have them map the development of neck tumors.	**Internet resources** The Voice Center at Eastern Virginia Medical School http://www.voice-center.com/laryngectomy.html Organization of Women Laryngectomy Survivors http://www.oowls.org/ International Association of Laryngectomies http://www.larynxlink.com/ WebWhispers http://www.webwhispers.org/ **Community resources** Have learners identify the number and type of resources available in their community for the client who needs speech rehabilitation.

7. Develop a teaching plan for the client who is getting ready to go home after undergoing a complete laryngectomy.	**Journaling** Describe the emotional responses to changes in body by the client and the family to head and neck cancer. Why is smoking cessation so difficult for the client? **Campus lab/Clinical component (25-30 min)** Demonstrate the appropriate techniques for suctioning and stoma care of the client undergoing a laryngectomy. **Numbered heads together (20-25 min)** Develop a teaching plan for assisting the client in speech rehabilitation. Have each group take a different approach. Give each group 10 minutes and then have them switch plans and provide additional information.	

Chapter 30: *Interventions for Clients with Noninfectious Lower Respiratory Problems*

Learning Outcomes	Learning Activities	Supplemental Resources
After reading this chapter, the student should be able to: 1. Explain the differences in pathophysiology between asthma and bronchoconstriction, and between asthma and inflammation. 2. Prioritize education needs for the client at step III of stepped therapy for asthma. 3. Interpret peak expiratory flow readings for the need for intervention. 4. Discuss the complications of long-term oral steroid therapy for treatment of chronic airflow limitations (CAL). 5. Compare and contrast the pathophysiology and clinical manifestations of asthma, bronchitis, and emphysema. 6. Identify risk factors for the development of chronic obstructive pulmonary disease. 7. Prioritize the education needs of the client with COPD who is receiving oxygen therapy at home.	**Group learning (5-10 min)** Assign learners to six groups. Provide each group the following vignette. Have groups members read and agree on answers to the questions. Have each group report on one question. Allow other groups to provide any additional information they may have regarding each question and answer presented. *Mr. Ralph Etterly, age 26, has just been admitted to the nursing unit complaining of severe chest pain, a frequent productive cough, and shortness of breath. A chest x-ray shows several large areas of dense infiltration over the lower lobes bilaterally. The laboratory has reported arterial blood gas values of pH, 7.36; Pao_2, 68; $Paco_2$, 55; and $PaHco_3$, 28.* 1. What is the priority problem for this client? 2. What led you to identify this problem? 3. What client outcome is desirable for this problem? 4. What nursing actions will help to achieve this outcome?	Worksheet 30-1 Worksheet 30-2 Worksheet 30-3 **Internet resources** American Lung Association http://www.lungusa.org/ National Heart, Lung, and Blood Institute, National Institutes of Health http://www.nhlbi.nih.gov/ American Academy of Allergy Asthma and Immunology. http://www.aaaai.org/ The National Emphysema Foundation http://emphysemafoundation.org/ Bronchitis http://www.healthylives.com/bronchitis.html

<table>
<tr>
<td>8. Describe interventions for energy conservation for the client with COPD.
9. Prioritize nursing care needs for the client immediately following lung volume reduction surgery.
10. Explain the nutritional requirements for the client with severe COPD.
11. Use laboratory data and clinical manifestations to determine the effectiveness of therapy for impaired gas exchange in a client with CAL.
12. Identify the risk factors that predispose to the development of lung cancer.
13. Compare and contrast the side effects of radiation treatment for lung cancer with those of chemotherapy for lung cancer.
14. Explain how to trouble shoot the chest tube drainage system in a client 1 day after a thoracotomy.</td>
<td>5. What do you think the physician will order for this client?
6. How will you know if your actions have helped?

Think-pair-share (3-5 min)
How do you think that incentive spirometry might change an ABG report?
How does the mechanism that controls the respiratory rate in the healthy individual compare with that of a person with CAL?
Provide the learners with the drug information worksheet (Worksheet 30-1) for learners to complete prior to class. Divide the learners into groups. Ask groups of learners to compare and contrast the various bronchodilators. In class, have each group present information regarding one drug class.
Provide the learners with the drug information worksheet (Worksheet 30-2) for learners to complete prior to class. Divide the learners into groups. Ask group learners to compare and contrast the various respiratory agents, expectorants, antitussives, and mucolytics. In class, have each group present information regarding one drug class.
What are the advantages of inhalation versus oral bronchodilators?
Why is the recommended diet for clients with CAL higher in fat calories rather than in carbohydrates?
What foods would be considered high fat but also require little energy to ingest (peanut butter, eggs, mayonnaise, fatty meats such as sausage, and salad dressings from corn, soy, and olive oil)?
Why can suction trigger cardiac dysrhythmias?</td>
<td>**Community resources**
Have groups of learners locate any community support groups such as “chronic lungers” for the client with COPD.</td>
</tr>
</table>

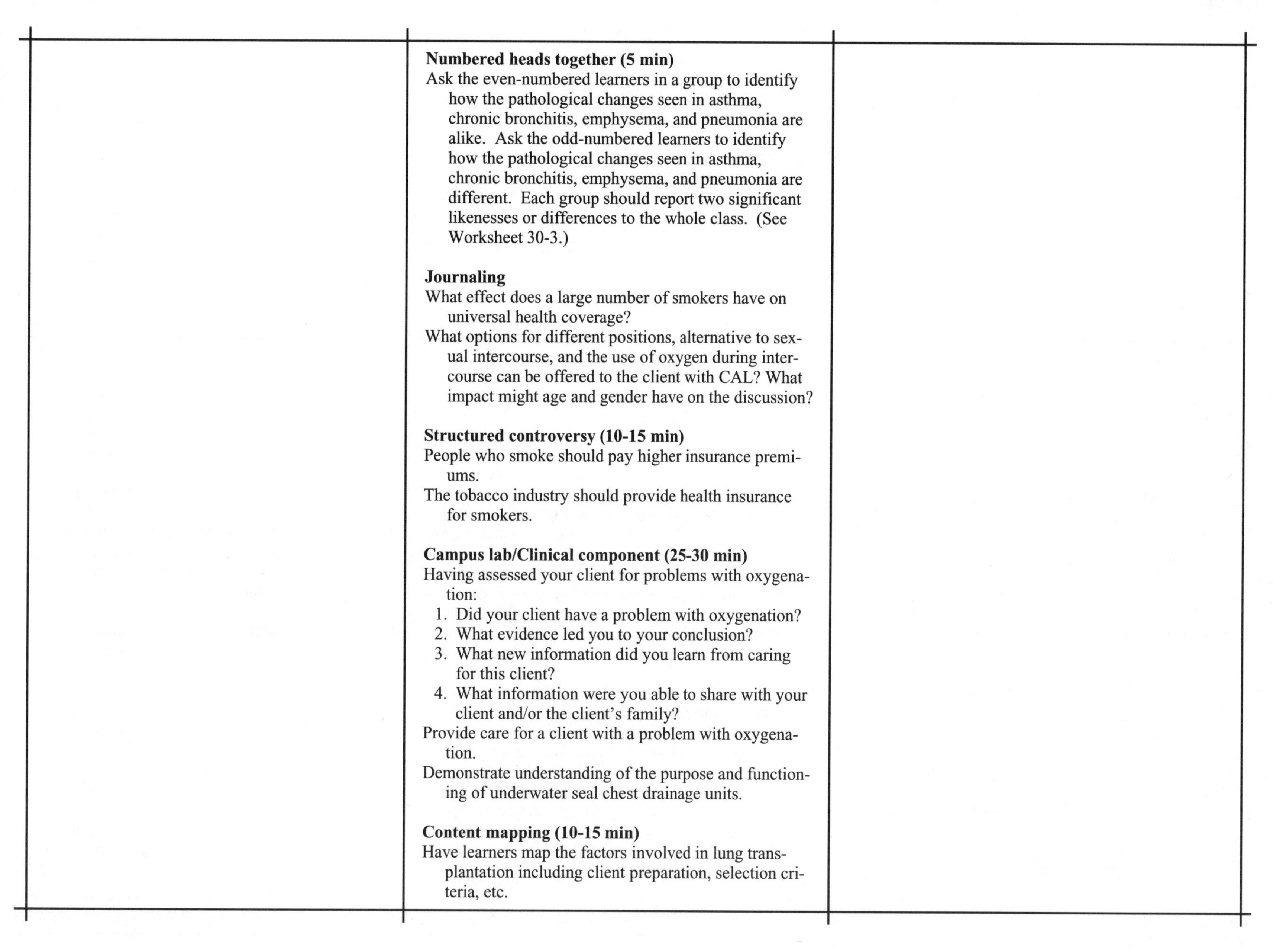

Numbered heads together (5 min)

Ask the even-numbered learners in a group to identify how the pathological changes seen in asthma, chronic bronchitis, emphysema, and pneumonia are alike. Ask the odd-numbered learners to identify how the pathological changes seen in asthma, chronic bronchitis, emphysema, and pneumonia are different. Each group should report two significant likenesses or differences to the whole class. (See Worksheet 30-3.)

Journaling

What effect does a large number of smokers have on universal health coverage?

What options for different positions, alternative to sexual intercourse, and the use of oxygen during intercourse can be offered to the client with CAL? What impact might age and gender have on the discussion?

Structured controversy (10-15 min)

People who smoke should pay higher insurance premiums.

The tobacco industry should provide health insurance for smokers.

Campus lab/Clinical component (25-30 min)

Having assessed your client for problems with oxygenation:

1. Did your client have a problem with oxygenation?
2. What evidence led you to your conclusion?
3. What new information did you learn from caring for this client?
4. What information were you able to share with your client and/or the client's family?

Provide care for a client with a problem with oxygenation.

Demonstrate understanding of the purpose and functioning of underwater seal chest drainage units.

Content mapping (10-15 min)

Have learners map the factors involved in lung transplantation including client preparation, selection criteria, etc.

Chapter 31: *Interventions for Clients with Infectious Respiratory Problems*

Learning Outcomes	Learning Activities	Supplemental Resources
After reading this chapter, the student should be able to: 1. Explain the consequences of an untreated streptococcal infection of the upper respiratory tract. 2. Identify adult populations at highest risk for contracting influenza. 3. Develop a teaching plan to prevent influenza in the older adult. 4. Identify clients at risk for developing community-acquired or hospital-acquired pneumonia. 5. Compare the clinical manifestations of pneumonia in the younger client with those exhibited by the older client with pneumonia. 6. Identify adult populations at risk for tuberculosis. 7. Interpret correctly the purified protein derivative test results for a person with normal immune function and a person with human immunodeficiency virus/acquired immunodeficiency syndrome. 8. Prioritize education needs for the client undergoing treatment at home for active tuberculosis.	**Think-pair-share (3-5 min)** Outside of etiology, what is the difference between allergic rhinitis and viral rhinitis? Why are clients undergoing transplants at increased risk for developing cytomegalovirus pneumonitis? What would the nurse expect to see on the chest x-ray of a client with pneumonia? Compare and contrast the diagnostic criteria confirming a diagnosis of tuberculosis. **Concept mapping (5-10 min)** Have learners map the clinical manifestations of pharyngitis. Have learners map the progression and resultant clinical manifestations of tuberculosis. **Journaling** Why should all older adults and individuals with a chronic illness receive annual pneumonia and influenza vaccinations?	**Internet resources** Pneumonia.net http://www.pneumonia.net/ Tuberculosis.net http://www.tuberculosis.net/ **Community resources** Where available, have groups of learners participate in influenza prevention and immunization clinics. Have groups of learners identify all resources available for influenza vaccines.

Chapter 32: *Interventions for Critically Ill Clients with Respiratory Problems*

Learning Outcomes	Learning Activities	Supplemental Resources
After reading this chapter, the student should be able to: 1. Identify clients at risk for development of pulmonary embolism. 2. Use laboratory data and clinical manifestations to determine the presence of acidosis. 3. Compare and contrast the ventilation-perfusion ratios for respiratory failure of ventilatory origin and respiratory failure of oxygenation origin. 4. Distinguish between normal and abnormal pulmonary capillary wedge pressure readings. 5. Use laboratory data and clinical manifestations to determine the adequacy of ventilatory interventions. 6. Describe the indications for intubation. 7. Prioritize nursing care needs for the conscious client being mechanically ventilated. 8. Identify clients at risk for development of pneumothorax.	**Think-pair-share (3-5 min)** Why are age and obesity risk factors for pulmonary embolism? Have learners identify client indicators that suggest that the client is ready to be weaned from the mechanical ventilation. Indicators include client is awake and has good muscle strength, has no life-threatening dysrhythmias, has clear chest sounds, and has a PaO_2 above 60 mm Hg when receiving 40% to 60% oxygen. Have learners identify interventions that are most likely to successfully wean the client who is ventilator dependent. A client undergoing mechanical ventilation is highly anxious and is fighting the ventilator. 1. What interventions are most likely to solve the problem? 2. What can you anticipate for negative reactions? 3. What are some of the ethical implications of the interventions you have suggested? Why are paralytic agents sometimes used in clients undergoing ventilation? Why are clients often taking heparin and warfarin sodium (Coumadin) at the same time? Why is malnutrition a problem in clients receiving mechanical ventilation? Why is flail chest considered an emergency situation? **Campus lab/Clinical component (25-30 min)** Correctly calculate a heparin infusion rate. Compare an INR with PTT and aPTT for the monitoring of heparin therapy. **Concept mapping (10-15 min)** Have learners map the relationship between the choice of ventilator type and client characteristics or disease process.	**Internet resources** Management of Deep Vein Thrombosis and Pulmonary Embolism http://www.americanheart.org/Scientific/statements/1996/069601.html **Community resources** What community resources are available to supply oxygen and home mechanical ventilators?

TM 28-1

OXYGEN DELIVERY SYSTEMS COMPARISON

Type	Advantages	Disadvantages
Low-flow delivery • Nasal cannula		
• Simple face mask		
• Partial rebreather		
• Nonrebreather		
High-flow delivery • Venturi		
• Other		
Transtracheal delivery		

TM 30-1

DRUG INFORMATION WORKSHEET

Bronchodilators

Drug/ Subclass	**Usual Dose/ Route**	**Expected Actions**	**Adverse Actions**	**Nursing Implications**
Sympathomimetics				
Methylxanthines				
Anticholinergics				
Corticosteroids				

TM 30-2

DRUG INFORMATION WORKSHEET

Antitussives, Expectorants, and Mucolytics

Drug/ Subclass	Usual Dose/ Route	Expected Actions	Adverse Actions	Nursing Implications
Antitussives				
Expectorants				
Mucolytics				

TM 30-3

SOME PATHOLOGICAL CONDITIONS THAT INTERFERE WITH GAS EXCHANGE

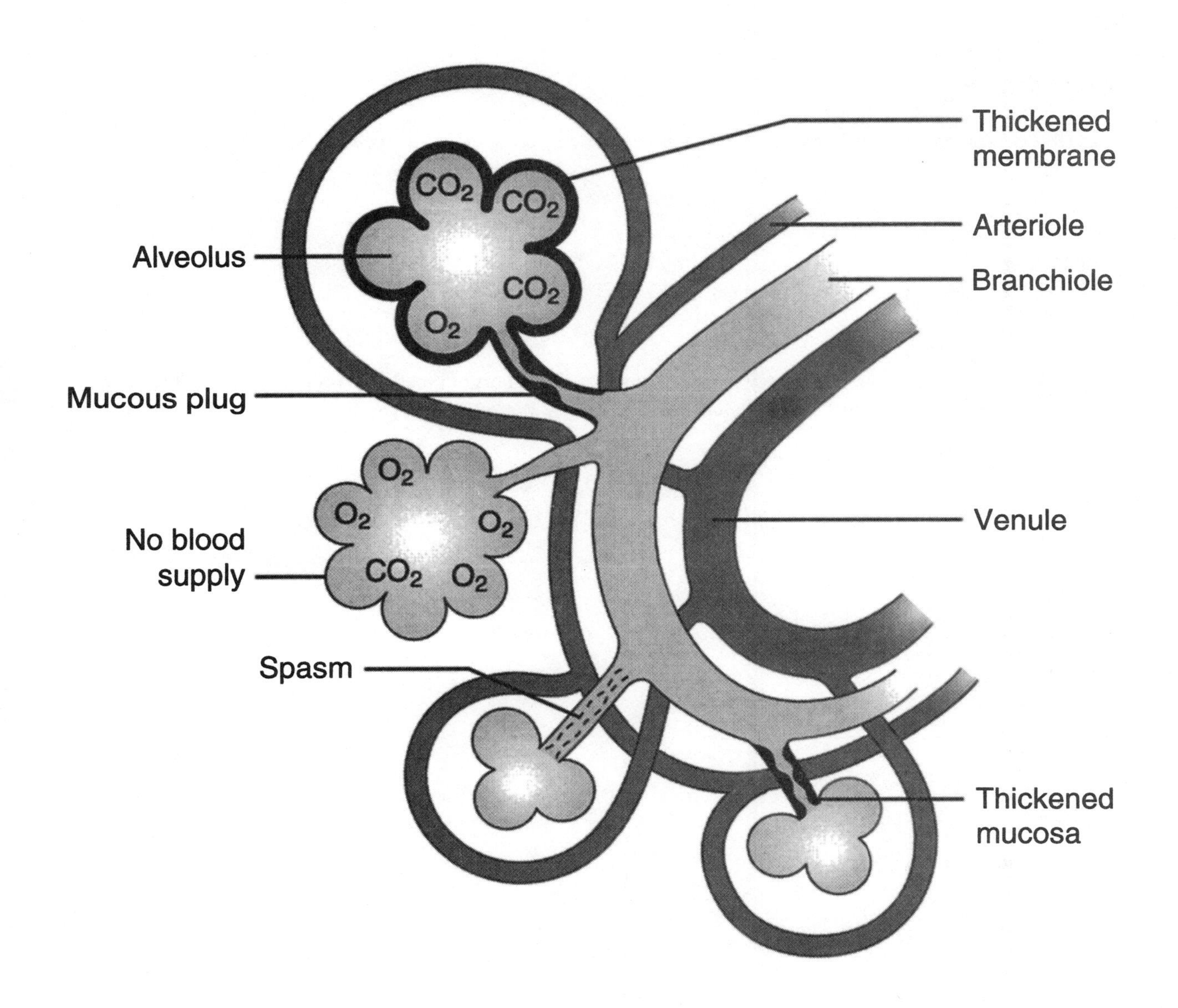

CHAPTER 28

Case Study for the Client Receiving Oxygen Therapy

A client has just returned from having an x-ray and put on his call light. You are in another client's room hanging an intravenous (IV) medication when the clerk who answered the light notifies you that the client said he was having some trouble breathing. The client has been receiving oxygen through nasal cannula at 2 L/min.

Questions

1. How do you decide whether you are going to complete hanging the IV medication before going to the client's room?

2. When you get to the client's room, you see that he is a little short of breath and proceed to check the oxygen equipment. What are you specifically checking for?

CHAPTER 29

Case Study for the Client with Vocal Cord Paralysis

You are making a home visit to a 64-year-old man with terminal lung cancer who is receiving hospice services at home. When you arrive, the client's wife tells you that she thinks he has a cold because his voice is hoarse and he has been coughing since breakfast, 20 minutes ago. On initial assessment, you find the client able to talk, but his voice is raspy and does not get louder with increased effort. He is somewhat anxious and says he is coughing because "some crumbs went down the wrong way." The color of his lips and nail beds is good. His respiratory rate and depth are within the range found at the last visit, 2 days ago.

Questions

1. What assessment information do you need to document?

2. What additional assessment data do you need to document?

3. What priority nursing actions do you need to implement?

4. What expected outcomes would be specific to this situation?

CHAPTER 30

Case Study for the Client with Chronic Obstructive Pulmonary Disease

A 55-year-old man arrives at your primary care clinic with complaints of persistent cough, shortness of breath, and occasional wheezing. His symptoms have become progressively worse over the past 2 weeks. The client's medical history includes hypertension. Social history includes tobacco use for 15 years, and the client currently smokes one pack of cigarettes per day.

Current medications include daily vitamins and atenolol, 50 mg/day. Vital signs are BP, 130/78; pulse, 96; and respirations, 26. The client denies any sputum production, fever, and chills.

Questions

1. While obtaining a history from your client, what important questions should you ask?

2. What initial physical assessments should you perform?

3. What are some possible diagnoses related to the symptoms?

4. What interventions may be ordered or implemented to minimize or treat the client's symptoms?

5. What are some key educational interventions related to health promotion or disease prevention that you will consider and/or implement?

CHAPTER 30

Case Study for the Client with Lung Cancer

A 62-year-old married man with three independent children was initially seen by his family physician and treated for an upper respiratory infection. His symptoms did not resolve, and further diagnostic tests were initiated. The client presents now with a 6-week history of right shoulder pain and dyspnea on exertion, cough productive of yellow sputum, a 7-pound weight loss over the last 4 weeks, and intermittent diaphoresis.

Medical History
No chronic illness
Pneumonia—1992
Bronchitis—"every year or so"
No current medications
Alcohol—social
Tobacco—quit smoking 4 years ago, prior 40-pack/y history

Family History
Father—deceased, aged 58 years, emphysema
Mother—deceased, aged 72 years, myocardial infarction
Brother—alive, aged 64 years, hypertension
Sisters—alive, aged 55, 56 years; no chronic illness

Physical Examination
Well-developed, alert and oriented male in no acute distress. Vital signs: afebrile, pulse, 124; respirations, 24; BP, 135/72. Neck examination revealed three right-sided supraclavicular lymph nodes measuring approximately 1 to 2 cm in diameter. Auscultation of the chest: lungs clear on the left and rhonchi on the right. The abdomen was soft, nondistended with positive bowel sounds in all quadrants and no hepatosplenomegaly. The extremities were without clubbing, cyanosis, or edema. Right shoulder and axilla tenderness was noted.

Diagnostic Studies
Chest CT revealed a 3-cm mass in the apex of the right lung with invasion into the right axilla. Additionally, tracheobronchial and mediastinal lymph node enlargement was noted. Bone scan results, normal; CT of head, mild atrophy without lesions; CT-guided fine-needle biopsy, tissue samples revealed adenocarcinoma of the lung, classified as non-small lung carcinoma; staging bronchoscopy and mediastonoscopy, bronchoscopy demonstrated no evidence of endobronchial lesions and mediastinoscopy additional mediastinal lymph node involvement measuring >1.5 cm; histological staging, stage IIIb, T2, N3, M0.

Questions

1. On the basis of the client's staging, what treatment is most likely to be recommended?

2. In preparing the client for treatment, what areas does the nurse need to include in the teaching plan?

3. What resources can the nurse direct the client to?

CHAPTER 31

*Case Study for the Client with Tuberculosis**

Your client is a 25-year-old inner-city woman with AIDS. She is hospitalized for active TB. She has four young children at home who are currently being cared for by her mother, a 42-year-old unemployed woman with diabetes mellitus.

Questions

1. What kind of isolation must the client be placed in and why?

2. Sputum cultures for AFB are ordered. When is the best time to collect sputum? Can you send sputum that contains saliva to the laboratory?

3. Before the client is discharged, what interventions need to be done at her home in preparation for her return?

*This Case Study is also available to students, along with web-based answer guidelines, in the *Critical Thinking Study Guide.*

CHAPTER 32

Case Study for the Client with ARDS

A 40-year-old man was exposed to toxic material in a manure bin during a farming accident that killed three other men. He inhaled CO_{21} ammonia gas, hydrogen sulfide, and methane gas, and he aspirated manure. The man was in the bin for an unknown period and when rescued, had no apparent respirations. A faint carotid pulse was palpated, so he was resuscitated, intubated, and transported to the hospital by helicopter, where x-ray showed bilateral diffuse infiltrates. His ABGs on 100% FIO_2 were pH, 7.25; $PaCO_2$, 40; and PaO_2, 40. His pulmonary shunt was calculated to be 35%.

Questions

1. What do the ABGs indicate about his oxygenation status?

2. For what treatment should you prepare?

3. He had large amount of frothy, bloody secretions suctioned from his endotracheal tube. The colloid osmotic pressure of the secretions was 19.0 and of his serum was 14.9. What does this indicate?

UNIT 7

PROBLEMS OF CARDIAC OUTPUT AND TISSUE PERFUSION: CARDIOVASCULAR SYSTEM

■ Core Concepts Grid

Anatomy	Physiology	Pathophysiology	History	Physical Exam	Diagnostic Tests	Interventions	Pharmacology
• **Heart chambers** • **Heart valves** • **Major vessels** • **Blood flow through the heart** • **Conduction system** SA node AV node His Bundle Purkinje fibers • **Peripheral vascular system** Arteries Arterioles Capillaries Venules Veins	• **Heart rate** • **Stroke volume** • **Cardiac output** • **Cardiac cycle** • **Blood pressure**	• **Hypertension** • **Infarction** • **Atherosclerosis** • **Pump failure** • **Inflammation** • **Hypertrophy** • **Infection/sepsis** • **Hypovolemia**	• **History of cardiac symptoms** • **Dyspnea** • **Fatigue** • **Paroxysmal nocturnal dyspnea** • **Orthopnea** • **Chest pain** • **Palpitations** • **Syncope** • **Cough** • **Past health history** • **Medications** • **Risk factors** Age Diet Activity Smoking	• **Cyanosis** • **Petechiae** • **Edema** • **Pulses** • **Heart sounds** S1-S4 • **Murmurs** • **Bruits** • **Blood pressure** • **Neck vein distention** • **Skin color** • **Hair distribution on extremities** • **Lesions** • **Clubbing** • **Dysrhythmias**	• **Chest x-ray** • **Electrocardiogram** • **Cardiac catheterization** • **Arteriography** • **Thallium scan** • **Exercise stress test** • **CK-MB** • **Lactate dehydrogenase** • **Cholesterol** • **Triglycerides** • **Lipoproteins** • **Myoglobin** • **Troponins** • **C-reactive protein**	• **Risk factor modification** • **Oxygen** • **Positioning** • **Pain control** • **Dysrhythmia monitoring** • **Diet modification** • **Heart transplantation** • **Coronary artery bypass graft (CABG)** • **MIDCAB** • **Percutaneous cardiac interventions (e.g., PTCA)** • **Fluid replacement** • **Hemodynamic monitoring** • **Mechanical ventilation** • **Cardiac rehabilitation** • **Health teaching**	• **Inotropic agent** • **Diuretics** • **Antidysrhythmics** • **Beta blockers** • **Vasodilators** • **Angiotensin-converting enzyme inhibitors** • **Calcium channel blockers** • **Nitrates** • **Anticoagulants** • **Antiplatelet agents** • **Morphine** • **Antibiotics** • **Antilipidemic agents**

Unit 7 (Chapters 33-38)

Problems of Cardiac Output and Tissue Perfusion: Management of Clients with Problems of the Cardiovascular System

Learning Plan

Chapter 33: *Assessment of the Cardiovascular System*

Learning Outcomes	Learning Activities	Supplemental Resources
After reading this chapter, the student should be able to: 1. Review the anatomy and physiology of the cardiovascular system. 2. Describe cardiovascular changes associated with aging. 3. Identify factors that place clients at risk for cardiovascular problems. 4. Perform appropriate assessments for clients with cardiovascular problems. 5. Interpret diagnostic test findings for clients with suspected or actual cardiovascular disease. 6. Explain the purpose of hemodynamic monitoring.	**Numbered heads together (5 min)** Ask even-numbered learners to list normal age-related changes in the cardiovascular system. Ask the odd-numbered learners to list changes in the cardiovascular system that are accelerated with elevation in serum cholesterol level, inactivity, and smoking. **Group learning** Ask groups of learners to list sequentially the sequence of blood flow through the heart to the body and return. Have them label all structures, including valves. Ask groups to draw the pathway of electrical activity during the cardiac cycle and to identify the timing intervals for the P-R interval, QRS wave, and Q-T interval. Ask learners to identify atrial and ventricular contraction in relation to the electrical activity they have identified. **Think-pair-share (3-5 min)** What factors of the autonomic nervous system control blood pressure? What is the association between a type A personality and risk of heart disease? What is preload and afterload? What factors might affect preload and afterload? What are the chances that a postmenopausal woman will have heart disease compared with a man of equal age and with other risk factors? What events produce gallops or murmurs? What is the role of homocysteine in cardiovascular disease?	**Internet resources** American Heart Association http://www.americanheart.org/ American Heart Association Council on Cardiovascular Nursing. http://www.americanheart.org/Scientific/council/cvn/ American Red Cross http://www.redcross.org/ National Heart Lung and Blood Institute http://www.nhlbi.nih.gov/ Cardiovascular Anatomy http://www.innerbody.com/image/cardov.html **Community resources** Have groups of learners attend a meeting of the local American Heart Association. Have groups of learners participate in a local "Jump for Heart."

	Campus lab/Clinical component (25-30 min) What cardiac risk factors did an assigned client have? What teaching can be planned to lower those risk factors? What is the probability that the client will change health behavior to lower the risk factors? What other strategies might increase the probability of compliance? What factors must be included to provide an accurate assessment of chest pain? Demonstrate a full cardiovascular assessment on one of your clients. After completing a cardiac assessment on an assigned client, assess any normal age-related changes to the cardiovascular system your client demonstrates. **Journaling** Until the early 1990s most cardiovascular research involved men. What probable differences in heart disease exist between men and women? What implications do those differences have on your cardiovascular assessments of men? Of women?	

Chapter 34: *Interventions for Clients with Dysrhythmias*

Learning Outcomes	Learning Activities	Supplemental Resources
After reading this chapter, the student should be able to: 1. Correlate the components of the electrocardiogram with the cardiac conduction system. 2. Interpret common cardiac dysrhythmias. 3. Identify typical assessment findings associated with common dysrhythmias. 4. Identify priority nursing diagnoses for clients experiencing dysrhythmias. 5. Plan care for clients experiencing common dysrhythmias. 6. Develop a teaching plan for clients experiencing common dysrhythmias. 7. Compare and contrast types of antidysrhythmic drugs.	**Group learning** Ask groups to draw the pathway of electrical activity during the cardiac cycle and to identify the timing intervals for the P-R interval, QRS wave, and Q-T interval. Ask learners to identify atrial and ventricular contraction in relation to the electrical activity they have identified. Obtain copies of rhythm strips demonstrating the more common rhythms and dysrhythmias (sinus bradycardia, sinus tachycardia, sinus dysrhythmia, PVC's, V-Tach, etc.). Give a set of strips to all learners. Have groups work together to identify the various rhythms. Let each group present findings on one rhythm at a time until all strips have been discussed. (Learners will need calipers for this exercise and the exercise may take up to 3 hours. The faculty member	Worksheet 34-1 **Audiovisuals** Essentials of Cardiac Rhythm Recognition by Medi-Sim, Williams & Wilkins, 1996. RxDx: Arrhythmias and Arrhythmias Tutorial, Part I and II., Lippincott, Williams & Wilkins, 1998.

8. Compare and contrast types of arterioventricular blocks.
9. Explain the purpose and types of pacing used as interventions for clients with dysrhythmias.
10. Outline the procedure and precautions associated with defibrillation.
11. Plan community-based care for a client after pacemaker or implantable cardioverter/defibrillator insertion.

could use the films or CD identified under additional resources.)

Have learner complete Worksheet 34-1 before coming to class. Divide learners into groups. Using the following vignettes and the information from Worksheet 34-1, have each group answer the following questions based on their vignette. At the conclusion have each group present the answers from their vignette.

1. What drug should you be prepared to administer?
2. What equipment is needed to administer this drug?
3. What contraindications should the nurse look for?
4. What assessments should be done first? Which, if any should be done on an ongoing basis? How frequently should they be done?
5. What do you think happened to this client? Why?

Vignette One:
Ms. Annette Bawker, 52, comes to the emergency department after she "fainted" twice at church. She is pail, her skin is cool and dry, and her pulse is 32.

Vignette Two:
Mrs. Henrietta Smith, 57, comes to the emergency department with a history of "indigestion" for 12 hours. She is weak and gray, and states she feels dizzy. The nurse performs a 12-lead ECG and has Mrs. Smith in semi-Fowler's position with oxygen at 5 L/min through a nasal cannula. Her vital signs are T= 97.6, P = 88, R = 24, and BP = 84/40. Mrs. Smith has no history of sudden severe fluid loss.

Vignette Three:
Mr. Harvey Dixon, 64, enters the emergency department complaining of severe chest pain lasting the last "hour or so." In addition to placing him in a semi-Fowler's position, putting on oxygen at 5 L min through a nasal cannula, and preparing morphine sulfate 4 to 8 mg IV by titration, you connect the ECG leads and get a 12-lead ECG. His ECG shows a run of five PVCs twice in 1 minute.

Vignette Four:
Mr. Charles Paquale, 76, enters the emergency department in asystole. You, the nurse, have little information about him.

Cardiac Monitoring: Basic, Series of 4 videos including: Basic Cardiac Monitoring; Understanding Fundamentals, Setting Up Cardiac Monitors, Dsyrhythmias of the SA Node and Atria and Dysrhythmias of the AV Node and Ventricles, Medcom.

The instructor should note that this is by no means an exhaustive list. A variety of programs and texts are available on this subject.

Internet resources
American Heart Association
http://www.americanheart.org/

American Heart Association Council on Cardiovascular Nursing
http://www.americanheart.org/Scientific/council/cvn/

American Red Cross
http://www.redcross.org/

National Heart, Lung, and Blood Institute
http://www.nhlbi.nih.gov/

Concept mapping (5-10 min)

Have learners map the changes in electrical conduction that occur with Atrial Fib/Flutter vs. First, Second, and Complete Heart Block vs. Ventricular Tachy/Fibrillation.

Think-pair-share (3-5 min)

How does a defibrillator work?

What is the difference between demand pacing and fixed rate pacing?

What are the possible complications of noninvasive temporary pacing?

What is the difference between cardioversion and defibrillation?

Campus lab/Clinical component (25-30 min)

Open a cardiac crash cart and identify the contents. Ask what the various drugs are used for during a code. Ask learners the roles of the various members of the code team. What is the code word for cardiac arrest at their particular facilities?

Approach a learner and tell him or her the client has just experienced a cardiac arrest. Ask the learner what he or she is going to do first, AFTER the learner calls for help.

Journaling

Until the early 1990s most cardiovascular research involved men. What probable differences in heart disease exist between men and women? What implications do those differences have on your cardiovascular assessments of men? Of women?

Structured controversy (10-15 min)

All clients who experience cardiac arrest should be resuscitated, even if they have a terminal illness.

Chapter 35: *Interventions for Clients with Cardiac Problems*

Learning Outcomes	Learning Activities	Supplemental Resources
After reading this chapter, the student should be able to: 1. Explain the pathophysiology of heart failure. 2. Compare and contrast left-sided and right-sided heart failure. 3. Perform a comprehensive assessment of clients experiencing heart failure. 4. Identify common nursing diagnoses and collaborative problems for clients with heart failure. 5. Evaluate the effects of interventions for reducing preload and afterload. 6. Describe special considerations for older adults with heart failure. 7. Discuss the prevention of complications for clients with heart failure. 8. Prioritize nursing care for clients experiencing heart failure. 9. Identify essential focused assessments used by the home health nurse for clients with heart failure. 10. Compare and contrast common valvular disorders. 11. Discuss surgical management for clients with valvular disease. 12. Develop a teaching/learning plan for clients with valvular disease. 13. Differentiate between common cardiac inflammations and infections—endocarditis, pericarditis, and rheumatic carditis. 14. Discuss the legal/ethical aspects related to heart transplantation, including cost of care.	**Concept mapping** Have learners concept map the pathophysiology of left-sided versus right-sided heart failure with associated signs and symptoms. **Group learning** Have groups of learners develop a day's meal plan for a client with a low-sodium diet, a low-caffeine diet, or a high-potassium diet. Have learners identify how the plan would need modification if the client was vegetarian, Hispanic, Jewish, or other. Have groups of learners identify how information about a client's fluid restriction plan can best be communicated among all health care providers. Include in the planning the best methods for communicating and monitoring the delegation of this task to unlicensed assistive personnel. Have each group develop a strategy for a client restricted to no more than 1500 mL per day and a plan for no more than 2000 mL per day. Ask learners to complete the worksheet on the classes of diuretics before class. After dividing into groups, have each group present information regarding one class, allowing time for all learners to add to their own chart. At the conclusion have each group discuss why a client might be taking more than one diuretic and identify the role of the nurse in monitoring an individual receiving these drugs (see Worksheet 35-1). **Think-pair-share (3-5 min)** Why is aging a factor in the development of heart failure? What impact do sympathomimetics have on the heart? What are the cardiac and noncardiac symptoms of digoxin toxicity? Why are some valvular disorders symptomatic and others asymptomatic? Why are individuals with valvular disorders often treated with prophylactic antibiotics prior to major surgical or dental events?	Worksheet 35-1 Worksheet 35-2 **Internet resources** American Heart Association http://www.americanheart.org/ American Heart Association Council on Cardiovascular Nursing http://www.americanheart.org/Scientific/council/cvn/ The Heart Failure Center http://www.heartcenteronline.com/myheartdr/Articles_about_the_heart/The_Heart_Failure_Center.html Heart Failure Society of America http://www.abouthf.org/

	What does the statement in your text, "The cause of pericarditis determines its presentation" mean? Give examples. What diet modifications might be necessary for the client with heart failure? **Numbered heads together (5 min)** Ask learners to complete the worksheet on the various valvular disorders before class. Ask groups of learners to identify the key nursing interventions for each of the disorders based on the physiology of the heart (see Worksheet 35-2). **Structured controversy (10-15 min)** Clients who have restrictive cardiomyopathy resulting from intravenous illicit drug use should be ineligible for heart transplantation.	

Chapter 36: *Interventions for Clients with Vascular Problems*

Learning Outcomes	Learning Activities	Supplemental Resources
After reading this chapter, the student should be able to: 1. Explain the pathophysiology of arteriosclerosis and atherosclerosis, including the factors that cause arterial injury. 2. Discuss the role of diet therapy in the management of clients with arteriosclerosis. 3. Describe the differences between essential and secondary hypertension. 4. Develop a plan of care for a client with essential hypertension. 5. Compare drug classifications used to treat hypertension. 6. Identify cultural considerations when caring for clients with hypertension. 7. Evaluate the effectiveness of interdisciplinary interventions to improve hypertension.	**Group learning (10-15 min)** Ask learners to draw the progression of atherosclerosis. Learners should be directed to identify the layers of the vessels as well as the elements involved in plaque formation. Then have them discuss the differences in vessel appearance between arteriosclerosis and atherosclerosis. Develop a 3-day diet plan for a step-one and a step-two diet plan to lower cholesterol. Ask learners to complete the worksheet on the various classifications of antihypertensive drugs before class. In class, ask different groups of learner to develop and present a decision for the use of vasodilators, calcium channel blockers, beta-blockers, diuretics and ACE inhibitors (see Worksheet 36-1). Draw the various forms of abdominal aortic aneurysms, including the involvement of arterial layers.	Worksheet 36-1 **Internet resources** National Heart Lung and Blood Institute http://www.nhlbi.nih.gov/ Hypertension Journal of the American Heart Association http://hyper.ahajournals.org/ Management of Deep Vein Thrombosis and Pulmonary Embolism http://www.americanheart.org/Scientific/statements/1996/069601.html **Community resources** Have groups of learners provide a blood pressure screening on campus.

8. Compare and contrast assessment findings typically present in clients with peripheral arterial and peripheral venous disease. 9. Prioritize postoperative care for clients who have undergone peripheral bypass surgery. 10. Develop a continuing plan for a client who has undergone an abdominal aortic aneurysm repair. 11. Compare and contrast Raynaud's disease and Berger's disease. 12. Describe the nurse's role in monitoring clients who are receiving anticoagulants, including unfractionated heparin, low molecular weight heparin, and warfarin.	Ask learners to compare arterial, venous, and diabetic ulcers. Ask each group of learners to defend the categories of comparison if selected. Ask a learner to write down all the different categories of comparison that the groups identify and to mark how many categories were the same in all groups. Ask each group to share the format they developed for making the comparison among types of ulcers. **Think-pair-share (3-5 min)** What is the role of homocysteine in the development of peripheral vascular disease? What is the relationship between hypertension and arteriosclerosis? Why is hypertension often called a "silent killer" disease? What is the role of the baroreceptors in the maintenance of blood pressure? Why is epistaxis often a sign of hypertension? What do the terms *inflow* and *outflow disease* mean in terms of signs and symptoms? What are the signs of graft occlusion/rupture? Why is paralytic ileus expected after aneurysm repair? What is the relationship between exposure to cold temperatures and Raynaud's disease? What is the relationship between smoking and Buerger's disease? What food should the client receiving warfarin avoid? What laboratory test monitors warfarin therapy? **Concept mapping (5-10 min)** Have learners draw a map of the renin-angiotensin-aldosterone system. As a portion of this assignment, have learners include in the map the site of actions of ACE inhibitor and angiotensin II receptor antagonist antihypertensive medications. **Numbered heads together** Have odd-numbered learners identify the cause and symptoms of PAD and have even-numbered learners identify the cause and symptoms of PVD. Make a general list for all learners to complete.	Have groups of learners provide a blood pressure screening in a local health fair.

Chapter 37: *Interventions for Clients in Shock*

Learning Outcomes	Learning Activities	Supplemental Resources
After reading this chapter, the student should be able to: 1. Describe the clinical manifestations associated with the compensatory mechanisms for shock. 2. Identify clients at risk for hypovolemic shock. 3. Use laboratory data and clinical manifestations to determine the effectiveness of therapy for shock. 4. Explain the basis for crystalloid versus colloid intravenous therapy for shock. 5. Prioritize nursing care needs for the client experiencing the nonprogressive stage of hypovolemic shock. 6. Compare and contrast the pathophysiology and clinical manifestations of the hyperdynamic and hypodynamic phases of septic shock. 7. Identify clients at risk for septic shock. 8. Develop an educational plan for prevention for the client at risk for septic shock who lives at home.	**Concept mapping** Ask groups of learners to map the fluid shifts and renal compensation during shock. Ask groups of learners to map the stages of shock according to pathophysiologic changes and client signs and symptoms. **Group learning** Ask groups of learners to complete the worksheet on hypovolemic, cardiogenic, obstructive, and distributive shock. Ask different groups of learners to identify essential clinical evidence for one type of shock, the priority interventions, and evaluation data that would indicate that the shock condition improved. Use Worksheet 37-1. Ask all learners to complete the worksheet comparing crystalloid and colloid agents for the treatment of shock. Divide the class into three groups. Ask one group to develop a decision tree for using fluids, one group to develop a tree for using blood or blood products, and one group to develop a tree for plasma expanders. Have each group be prepared to report on the major considerations for the use of each product. Use Worksheet 37-2. **Think-pair-share (3-5 min)** What is the relationship between histamine and anaphylaxis? What mechanism does the renal system use as a compensatory mechanism in hypovolemic shock? **Journaling** What liability is assumed by the health care team if a client develops a blood-borne infection while receiving a transfusion in a shock situation?	**Internet resources** Worksheet 37-1 Worksheet 37-2 Hypovolemic Shock: Is your patient at risk? http://www.springnet.com/ce/p509a.htm Emergency Medicine: Shock http://www.vh.org/Providers/ClinRef/FPHandbook/Chapter01/18-1.html

Chapter 38: *Interventions for Critically Ill Clients with Coronary Artery Disease*

Learning Outcomes	Learning Activities	Supplemental Resources
After reading this chapter, the student should be able to: 1. Explain the pathophysiology of coronary artery disease (CAD). 2. Compare and contrast stable angina, unstable angina, and myocardial infarction (MI). 3. Identify modifiable and nonmodifiable risk factors for CAD. 4. Interpret physical and diagnostic assessment findings in clients who have CAD. 5. Describe the psychosocial aspects of CAD. 6. Prioritize care for clients who have CAD. 7. Explain the advantages of thrombolysis for a client experiencing an MI. 8. Identify the life-threatening complications of CAD. 9. Describe the postoperative care for the client who has undergone coronary artery bypass graft (CABG) surgery. 10. Discuss the differences among CABG surgery, minimally invasive direct coronary artery bypass, and transmyocardial laser revascularization. 11. Develop a discharge plan for the client with CAD.	**Concept mapping** Ask groups of learners to map the ECG changes associated with myocardial ischemia, injury, and infarction. **Think-pair-share (3-5 min)** Describe the concept of a "silent heart attack." How can the presence of client hostility and mistrust predict a heart attack? How might a client with an implantable defibrillation device (ICD) become a "no-code"? How does nitroglycerin diminish the pain of angina? What is the role of aspirin in the prevention of heart disease and in decreasing the severity of a myocardial infarction (MI)? Does aspirin work as well for women as for men? What impact does cocaine have on the heart? Why is sodium bicarbonate used during a code situation? Why do women have higher morbidity and mortality rates after MI than men? Why is morphine sulfate a good drug of choice to treat the pain of MI? What does the use of an intraaortic balloon pump promote in the patient with cardiogenic shock? **Numbered heads together (5-10 min)** Ask even-numbered heads to develop a list of priority assessments and interventions for the client receiving thrombolytic therapy for an acute myocardial infarction in the emergency department. Ask the odd-numbered learners to develop a list of priority assessments and interventions for the client receiving thromboytic therapy for an acute myocardial infarction in the 4- to 12-hour period following thrombolytic therapy. Each group should be asked to identify the essential client symptoms of complications for the therapy.	**Internet resources** The Heart Attack Center http://www.heartcenteronline.com/ The Mended Hearts, Inc. http://www.mendedhearts.org/ MedicineNet.com: Heart Attack http://www.medicinenet.com/Script/Main/art.asp?articlekey=379 Heart Information Network http://www.heartinfo.org/hrtatkang.html The Bypass Surgery Center http://www.heartcenteronline.com/myheartdr/Articles_about_the_heart/The_Bypass_Surgery_Center.html **Community resources** Have groups of learners contact the American Heart Association and determine what material is available regarding risk factors. Have learners become CPR certified.

	Concept mapping Have learners map the differences and similarities between the use of percutaneous coronary angioplasty, stent placement, and CABG. **Journaling** Why do MI clients often feel a “sense of doom, and what are the nursing responsibilities in this response? **Structured controversy** What should become of clients who Medicare determines should not be candidates for CABG intervention? Clients who continue to smoke, fail to lose weight, and are unable to control their cholesterol levels should not be candidates for CABG intervention. **Campus laboratory/Clinical component** Role play the conversation between a nurse and a client, both male and female, regarding the resumption of sexual activity after MI.	

TM 34-1

CARDIAC EMERGENCY DRUGS

Drug	Action	Indications for Use	Side/ Adverse Effects	Indications
Lidocaine				
Epinephrine				
Atropine				
Dopamine				

TM 35-1

DIURETIC DRUG COMPARISONS

Drug	Acts Where in Nephron?	Indication for Use	Side/Adverse Effects	Implications
Carbonic anhydrase Inhibitors Acetazolamide (Diamox)				
Loop diuretics Furosemide (Lasix) Ethacrynic acid (Edecrin)				
Thiazide and thiazide-like diuretics Chlorothiazide Metolazone (Zaroxolyn)				
Potassium-sparing diuretics Triamterene (Dyrenium) Spironolactone (Aldactone)				

TM 35-2

VALVULAR DISORDERS

	Pathophysiology	Symptoms
Mitral stenosis		
Mitral insufficiency		
Mitral valve prolapse		
Aortic stenosis		
Aortic insufficiency		

TM 36-1

ANTIHYPERTENSIVE DRUGS COMPARISON

Drug Class	Action	Usual Dose/ Route	Side/Adverse Effects
Vasodilators Hydralazine (Apresoline)			
Beta-adrenergic blocking agents Propanolol (Inderal) Atenolol (Tenormin)			
Diuretics Furosemide (Lasix) Spironolactone (Aldactone)			
Calcium channel blockers Nifedipine (Procardia) Verapamil (Calan)			
Angiotensin-converting enzyme inhibitors Captoril (Capoten)			
Angiotensin II receptor blockers Losartan (Cozaar)			

TM 37-1

SHOCK COMPARISON

Type of Shock	Causes	Pathophysiology	Signs/Symptoms
Hypovolemic			
Cardiogenic			
Distributive			
Obstructive			

TM 37-2

SHOCK FLUID THERAPY

Type of Product	Indications for Use	Usual Dosage	Nursing Implications
Blood and blood products Whole blood Packed red blood cells Albumin			
Plasma expanders Hydroxyethyl starch (Hetastarch) Dextran Mannitol			
Crystalloids Normal saline Ringer's solution 5% dextrose in water			

CHAPTER 35

Case Study for the Client with Heart Failure

An 85-year-old female client is a nursing home resident. She has a long history of heart failure, myocardial infarction, pulmonary emphysema, hypertension, and degenerative joint disease. Her medications include: Lasix 20 mg QD, Vasotec 5 mg QD, digoxin 0.125 mg QD, KCl 40 mEq QD, and Motrin 200 mg QID.

Today she complains that she "just doesn't feel right." The nursing assistant reports that the resident's pulse is weak and irregular at 116 BPM, and her skin feels cooler than usual. You go to her room for further assessment.

Questions

1. When taking a history from this client, what important questions would you ask?

2. What physical assessment techniques would you perform?

3. During the assessment, you find that she is dyspneic at rest, has a respiratory rate of 32, has a BP of 180/95, is very anxious, and has crackles in the bases of her lungs. What should you do first?

CHAPTER 37

*Case Study for the Client with Hypovolemic Shock**

A 38-year-old female client returned to the postanesthesia recovery area 2 hours ago, after undergoing a tubal ligation by colposcopy (through the back wall of the vagina behind the cervix). Her last documented vital signs, taken 30 minutes ago, were BP = 102/80, pulse = 88, and respirations = 22. You now note that her face is pale, and the skin around her lips has a bluish cast. Her vital signs are now: BP = 90/76, P = 98, and respirations = 28.

Questions

1. What additional assessment techniques would you perform?

2. Where would you look for hemorrhage?

3. What other data would you gather?

4. When you reassess her in 15 minutes, you find the following vital signs: BP = 88/70, pulse = 102, and respirations = 30. She wakes when you shake her arm and complains of back pain and thirst. Given these findings, what are your action priorities?

5. What expected outcomes would be specific to this situation?

*This Case Study is also available to students, along with web-based answer guidelines, in the *Critical Thinking Study Guide.*

UNIT 8 PROBLEMS OF TISSUE PERFUSION: HEMATOLOGIC SYSTEM ■ Core Concepts Grid

Anatomy	Physiology	Pathophysiology	History	Physical Exam	Diagnostic Tests	Interventions	Pharmacology
• Blood cells • Plasma • Lymph system • Bone marrow	• Oxygen transport • Hematopoe-sis • Phagocytosis • Blood-clotting mechanism	• Hemolysis • Insufficient pro-duction • Hyperproduction • Active loss • Defective cells • Hypoxia • Hypoxemia	• History of bleeding • Fatigue • Bruising • Weakness • Weight loss • Behavioral changes • Anorexia	• Bruising • Pallor • Tachycardia • Tachypnea • Hypotension • Pain • Swelling • Purpura • Infection • Decreased level of con-sciousness • Skin ulcers • Jaundice • Glossitis • Paresthesias	• Hemoglobin • Hematocrit • Red blood cell count (RBC) • White blood cell count (WBC) • Platelet count • Erythrocyte sedimentation rate (ESR) • WBC differential • Prothrombin time (PT) • Partial thrombo-plastin time (PTT) • Activated partial thromboplastic time (aPPT) • International Normalized Ratio (INR) • Bone marrow biopsy • Iron	• Blood transfusions • Phlebotomy • Radiation • Chemotherapy • Diet modification • Pain control • Fluids (oral and parenteral) • Bone marrow transplantation • Bleeding precautions • Energy conservation • Health teaching	• Iron supplements • Chemotherapy • Anticoagulants • Opioids • Antivirals • Antifungals • Antibiotics

Unit 8 (Chapters 39-40)

Problems of Tissue Perfusion: Management of Clients with Problems of the Hematologic System

Learning Plan

Chapter 39: *Assessment of the Hematologic System*

Learning Outcomes	Learning Activities	Supplemental Resources
After studying this chapter, the student should be able to: 1. Describe hematologic changes associated with aging. 2. Explain the process of erythrocyte maturation. 3. Describe the role of platelets in hemostasis. 4. Compare and contrast the structure and function of platelet plugs and fibrin clots. 5. Interpret blood cell counts and clotting tests to assess the client's hematologic status. 6. Compare and contrast the actions and uses of anticoagulants and thrombolytics. 7. Prioritize nursing care for the client after bone marrow aspiration.	**Think-pair-share (3-5 min)** What are the normal age-related changes in blood counts? Ask groups of learners to diagram the process of hemostasis. Ask groups of learners to list the steps involved in blood specimen collection. Make a chart of commonly used anticoagulants and thrombolytic agents, their antidotes (if appropriate) and the lab tests that monitor their effectiveness. How can serum albumin, total protein, total iron binding capacity (TIBC), or immunoglobulin levels be used to indicate nutritional status? **Journaling (15-30 min)** Have learners examine OSHA safety standards—with respect to blood—in a clinical setting and document findings. Document the observation of a bone marrow aspiration. How does the donor react? How is the bone marrow handled and stored? **Concept mapping (10-15 min)** Map the maturation process of the three cellular blood components. Diagram the cascade of coagulation.	**Internet resources** American Red Cross http://www.redcross.org/ National Heart, Lung, and Blood Institute http://www.nhlbi.nih.gov/ American Society of Hematology http://www.hematology.org/ Understanding von Willebrand Disease http://www.wfh.org/von_w.html **Community resources** Invite a phlebotomist/lab technician to discuss how tests are carried out in the laboratory. Have learners list the risks – both on the accuracy of reporting as well as to the employees. Visit a bone marrow bank to investigate screening and protocols. Have learners complete a community assessment of the percentage of the local population who have volunteered to be donors. Obtain materials form the local chapter of the American Cancer Society on the prediction of mortality and frequency of cancer for the upcoming year. Supply as a handout to the class.

Chapter 40: *Interventions for Clients with Hematologic Problems*

Learning Outcomes	Learning Activities	Supplemental Resources
After studying this chapter, the student should be able to: 1. Identify three clinical manifestations common to clients who have any type of anemia. 2. Explain the pattern of inheritance for sickle cell disease. 3. Prioritize nursing care needs for the client who has sickle cell disease. 4. Plan a diet for a client who has iron deficiency anemia or vitamin B_{12} deficiency anemia. 5. Explain the mechanism of action and potential side effects of epoetin alpha therapy. 6. Compare and contrast the pathologic mechanisms of hemolytic anemia versus aplastic anemia. 7. Compare and contrast leukemia and lymphoma for etiology, pathophysiology, and clinical manifestations. 8. List four risk factors for the development of leukemia. 9. Analyze laboratory data and clinical manifestations to determine the presence of infection in a client who has neutropenia. 10. Compare the purposes and scheduling of induction therapy, consolidation therapy, and maintenance therapy for leukemia. 11. Prioritize nursing interventions for the client with neutropenia. 12. Prioritize nursing interventions for the client with thrombocytopenia. 13. Develop a teaching plan for a client with thrombocytopenia who is at home. 14. Prioritize nursing responsibilities during transfusion therapy. 15. Identify clients at risk for complications of transfusion therapy.	**Think-pair-share (3-5 min)** Have learners complete TM 40-1 prior to class; compare answers. What type of blood product would be appropriate for various types of anemias and blood problems? Have learners complete TM 40-2 prior to class; compare answers. Identify and prioritize interventions for each type of reaction. What might a fissured tongue indicate? How does immunoglobulin therapy help a client with severe immunodeficiency problems? Explain the benefits of autologous blood donation. Ask groups of learners to diagram the process of blood transfusion. Include safety checks and the sequence of assessments during the transfusion. **Pairs check (10-15 min)** Role-play a transfusion scenario—from the recipient being typed and screened to the nurse's retrieving blood from the blood bank and starting the transfusion. Document. **Concept mapping (10-15 min)** Map the concepts of blood typing and matching and include universal donor and recipient. **Numbered heads together (3-5 min)** Ask even-numbered learners to identify assessments of normal oral mucosa, both subjective and objective. Ask odd-numbered learners to identify the impact of chemotherapy on oral mucosa and the assessments that would confirm stomatitis.	**Transparency masters** TM 40-1 Comparison of blood components TM 40-2 Comparison of blood transfusion reactions **Internet resources** American Association of Blood Banks http://www.aabb.org/ International Association of Sickle Cell Nurses and Physician Assistants http://www.emory.edu/PEDS/SICKLE/parnpage.htm National Hemophilia Foundation http://www.hemophilia.org/home.htm Anemia: An approach to Diagnosis http://www.ohsu.edu/som-hemonc/handouts/deloughery/anemia.shtml The Leukemia & Lymphoma Society http://www.leukemia.org/hm_lls Glossary of Lymphoma Terms http://www.lymphomainfo.net/lymphoma/glossary.html **Community resources** Local or state chapter of: • American Cancer Society • American Hemophilia Society • American Society of Hematology • American Red Cross Invite a representative from the American Red Cross to discuss blood collection, screening, storage and distribution. Arrange for learners to help with a blood drive, if possible.

<table>
<tr>
<td></td>
<td>Ask different groups of learners to list the clinical assessments that would confirm an oncological emergency—septicemia, disseminated intravascular coagulation, hypercalcemia or superior vena cava syndrome (SVCS). Switch lists among groups. After verifying the lists, have each group develop a list of interventions that would improve listed symptoms. Switch lists again. Have groups prioritize listed interventions. The groups should also identify which interventions may be done by the RN, the LPN/LVN or delegated to unlicensed assistive personnel (UAP).
Have learners construct a day's worth of menus for a client with anemia. Ask them to pay particular attention to cultural or ethnic food preferences.

Send a problem (10-15 min)
Have learners write a test review question on bone marrow transplantation in clients with leukemia. Focus on the client's immunosuppressed status.

Structured controversy (10-15 min)
Is it unethical not to offer experimental drugs to clients for whom other treatments have been unsuccessful?

Structured controversy (15-20 min)
Has the incidence of HIV increased in populations that require frequent use of blood and blood products, such as hemophiliacs?</td>
<td>Interview an individual who is experiencing a chronic blood problem. Document methods used (past and present) to treat the problem.

Examine educational material available from the American Cancer Society regarding safe handling of toxic and carcinogenic agents.</td>
</tr>
</table>

TM 40-1

COMPARISON OF BLOOD COMPONENTS

Component	Indications for Use	Potential Adverse Effects
Packed red blood cells		
Washed red blood cells		
Platelets		
Fresh frozen platelets		
Cryoprecipitate		
White blood cells		

American Association of Blood Banks (AABB) has excellent online information.

TM 40-2

COMPARISON OF TRANSFUSION REACTIONS

Type of Reaction	Signs/Symptoms	When Likely	Nursing Interventions
Hemolytic			
Allergic			
Febrile			
Bacterial			
Overload			

UNIT 9 PROBLEMS OF MOBILITY, SENSATION, AND COGNITION: NERVOUS SYSTEM ■ Core Concepts Grid

Anatomy	Physiology	Pathophysiology	History	Physical Exam	Diagnostic Tests	Interventions	Pharmacology
• **Central system** Brain Cerebrum Cerebellum Limbic system Brainstem Reticular activating system (RAS) Spinal cord Meninges Ventricles Sensory pathways Motor pathways Reflex arcs • **Peripheral system** Cranial nerves Autonomic nervous system	• **Coordination** Movement Equilibrium • **Regulation** • **Mental activity** Consciousness Memory Thinking • **Nerve impulse** Transmission • **Sensation**	• **Infection** • **Inflammation** • **Obstruction** • **Seizure activity** • **Paralysis** • **Paresis** • **Fasciculations** • **Increased intracranial pressure (ICP)** • **Bradykinesia** • **Tremors** • **Hemorrhage** • **Ischemia** • **Plaques and tangles** • **Tumors**	• **Past history of neurologic symptoms** • **Past history of neurologic trauma, infections** • **Family history** Familial neurologic diseases • **Social history** Drugs Occupation Age	• **Mental status** General appearance Orientation Mood/affect Thought content Intelligence Recent/remote memory • **Cranial nerves** • **Motor system** Muscles Balance Coordinated movement • **Sensory system** Light touch Pain Temperature Vibration Position Recognition • **Reflexes** • **Other** Romberg's test Brudzinski's sign Kernig's sign • **Functional assessment** • **Speech and language ability**	• **Radiologic** Skull, spine Computed tomography (CT) • **Magnetic resonance imaging (MRI)** • **Electroencephalogram (EEG)** • **Lumbar puncture (LP)** • **Cerebrospinal fluid** • **Toxic drug –levels**	• **Environmental modification** Quiet Dim light Padded rails • **Bladder training** • **Bowel training** • **Positioning** • **Nutrition** • **Airway management** • **Lifestyle modification** • **Imunosuppressive therapy** • **Intracranial pressure (ICP) monitoring** • **Rehabilitation (physical and vocational)**	• **Anticonvulsants** • **Antispasmotics** • **Dopaminergics** • **Anticholinergics** • **Dopamine agonists** • **Anti-cholinesterases** • **Antibiotics** • **Cholinergics**

Unit 9 (Chapters 41-45)

Problems of Mobility, Sensation, and Cognition: Management of Clients with Problems of the Nervous System

Learning Plan

Chapter 41: *Assessment of the Nervous System*

Learning Outcomes	Learning Activities	Supplemental Resources
After reading this chapter, the student should be able to: 1. Explain the function of the major divisions of the nervous system. 2. Identify common physiologic changes associated with aging that affect the nervous system. 3. Perform a neurologic history based on Gordon's functional health patterns. 4. Perform a basic neurologic physical assessment. 5. Perform a rapid neurologic assessment. 6. Plan pretest and follow-up care for clients undergoing common neurologic diagnostic tests.	**Think-pair-share (3-5 min)** Describe the "fight or flight" response as a lifesaving process. Identify the purpose and significance of the reflexes in the body. Differentiate the functions of the anterior and posterior spinal tracts. Identify the essential elements for documenting a neurological assessment. What factors affect neurotransmission? What important properties does the blood-brain barrier possess? Discuss the clinical significance of Romberg's test, Brudzinski's sign and Kernig's sign. Identify the advantages and disadvantages of a lumbar puncture. Compare the procedure and care for clients undergoing a lumbar puncture and myelography. **Concept mapping (5-10 min)** Ask learners to map the major parts of the brain, including the cerebrum, cerebellum, diencephalon, and brainstem. **Pairs check (10 -15 min)** Have learners perform a mini-mental status examination (MMSE) on each other. Have learners demonstrate the Glascow Coma Scale examination on each other. **Campus lab/Clinical component (10-15 min)** Have learners perform an MMSE on any client and submit for review. Demonstrate the patient preparation necessary for an electroencephalograph (EEG).	**Internet resources** Neurologic Examination http://www.medinfo.ufl.edu/year1/bcs/clist/neuro.html

	Journaling Discuss how the cognitive changes of aging might affect mental status.	

Chapter 42: *Interventions for Clients with Problems of the Central Nervous System: The Brain*

Learning Outcomes	Learning Activities	Supplemental Resources
After reading this chapter, the student should be able to: 1. Compare migraine and cluster headaches in terms of assessment findings. 2. Develop a teaching plan for a client diagnosed with migraine headaches. 3. Differentiate the common types of seizures, including presenting clinical manifestations and management. 4. Explain the nurse's role in implementing seizure precautions. 5. Plan and document care for a client experiencing a seizure. 6. Identify collaborative management options for treating clients diagnosed with epilepsy. 7. Outline the priorities for care of clients with meningitis and encephalitis. 8. Describe the pathophysiology of Parkinson's disease. 9. Develop a community-based plan of care for a client with Parkinson's disease. 10. Outline realistic expected outcomes for clients with Alzheimer's disease. 11. Explain the use of drug therapy for clients with Alzheimer's disease. 12. Develop a teaching plan for caregivers of clients with Alzheimer's disease in community-based settings.	**Think-pair-share (3-5 min)** Identify nutritional triggers for the client with migraine headaches. Compare and contrast the pharmacological agents used to prevent and treat clients with migraine headaches. Describe what adaptations might be necessary when teaching older adult clients. Describe seizure precautions. Identify essential elements of documentation for a client experiencing a seizure. Describe the client in the late stages of Parkinson's disease. List nursing diagnoses for the client with advanced Parkinson's disease. Identify individuals most at risk for developing dementia. Discuss the purpose of drug therapy for clients with Alzheimer's disease. What are the long-term effects of levodopa? What are the similarities and differences between and among CNS infections—encephalitis, meningitis, and Creutzfeldt-Jakob disease? Why might college or university officials be concerned about one or two cases of meningitis among their students? **Concept mapping (5-10 min)** Have learners draw a concept map of the treatment of status epilpeticus.	Worksheet 42-1 **Internet resources** Alzheimer's Association http://www.alz.org/ Epilepsy Foundation http://www.efa.org/ Epilepsy Ontario http://epilepsyontario.org/ Huntington's Disease Society of America http://www.hdsa.org/ American Council for Headache Education http://www.achenet.org/ The National Migraine Association http://www.migraines.org/ National Headache Foundation http://www.headaches.org/ Migraine Information Center http://www.ama-assn.org/special/migraine/migraine.htm National Parkinson Foundation Incorporated http://www.parkinson.org/

	Pairs check (10-15 min) Have pairs of learners develop a decision tree of the selection of medications used in the treatment of Parkinson's disease. **Campus lab/Clinical component** Evaluate your client for any symptoms of Parkinson's disease. Be prepared to discuss medications that carry side effects that mirror Parkinson's disease. **Journaling** What therapeutic communication skills were used when caring for the client with dementia? What psychosocial struggles are encountered by the family of an Alzheimer's client? What would you teach the client's family regarding the safety needs of the client with Alzheimer's disease? **Group learning (20-30 min)** Have groups of learners complete Worksheet 42-1, Nursing Interventions for Clients with Alzheimer's Disease. Have one group provide answers for Stage I, the next group for Stage II, etc. Allow all learners to provide additional answers for the entire group. Divide the class into groups of four or five and have them map common concepts for the care of clients during each stage of Alzheimer's disease. **Structured controversy (10-15 min)** Should fetal tissue transplants be used in the treatment of Parkinson's disease? Should clients with seizure disorders be allowed to drive a car? Have students research the laws in their state. Should demented clients in a nursing home be placed in a specialty dementia unit or be integrated with other residents? Should families with a history of Huntington's disease be required to have genetic counseling. If the genetic marker is found, what should the family be told? Should clients with late-stage Alzheimer's disease who are not eating be fed?	The Parkinson's Institute http://www.parkinsonsinstitute.org/ The American Parkinsons Disease Association, Inc. http://apdaparkinson.com/ **Community resources** Have groups of learners determine what support groups are available in their community for clients with Parkinson's and Alzheimer's Disease. Have groups of learners determine the availability of respite programs for families of clients with Alzheimer's and Parkinson's disease clients. Invite a nurse working in a headache clinic to discuss care for clients with varying types of headaches.

Chapter 43: *Interventions for Clients with Problems of the Central Nervous System: The Spinal Cord*

Learning Outcomes	Learning Activities	Supplemental Resources
After reading this chapter, the student should be able to: 1. Identify risk factors that contribute to back pain. 2. Explain ways to prevent back pain. 3. Plan care for the client having a diskectomy, laminectomy, and/or spinal fusion. 4. Analyze the common nursing diagnoses and collaborative problem for the client with an acute spinal cord injury (SCI). 5. Describe typical medical complications that are experienced by clients with an SCI. 6. Prioritize care for the client with an SCI. 7. State the expected outcomes for the client with an SCI. 8. Develop a community-based teaching plan for clients who have an SCI. 9. Identify the clinical manifestations associated with spinal cord tumors. 10. Explain the pathophysiology of multiple sclerosis (MS), including the six basic types. 11. Discuss the role of medications in treating clients with MS. 12. Develop a community-based teaching plan for a client with MS. 13. Compare and contrast the clinical manifestations of MS and amyotrophic lateral sclerosis.	**Group learning** Have groups of learners work together to complete Worksheet 43-1. When groups appear near finishing have each group give their sheet to the next group and fill in any additional information the group might have. Make enough copies for all groups to have completed sheets. Have groups of learners differentiate the care of an SCI client in the "field" and in the rehabilitation unit. **Think-pair-share (3-5 min)** What is the difference between a diskectomy and a laminectomy in the clients' recovery time? What is failed back surgery syndrome (FBSS)? Identify risk factors for clients with head and SCI. Who is most likely to have traumatic CNS injury? Describe body image changes that occur following an SCI. Identify lifestyle alterations necessary for clients who are paraplegic or quadriplegic. Discuss the sexual and erectile dysfunction of the client with SCI. Discuss the quality of life for clients with chronic back pain. What is postpolio syndrome, and why does it occur? Identify the pathophysiology of spinal shock. What diagnostic tests may help differentiate multiple sclerosis from a spinal tumor? What is the rationale for considering multiple sclerosis as an autoimmune disease? **Concept mapping** Have learners develop a map demonstrating the signs and symptoms associated with the various levels of SCI. Have learners develop a map detailing the six types of MS according to clinical manifestations.	Worksheet 43-1 **Internet resources** Christopher Reeve Paralysis Foundation http://apacure.com/ Spinal Cord Injury Resource Center http://www.spinalinjury.net/ National Spinal Cord Injury Association http://www.spinalcord.org/ International Spinal Development & Research Foundation http://www.spine-research.org/ National Multiple Sclerosis Society http://www.nmss.org/ The Multiple Sclerosis Foundation http://www.msfacts.org/ International MS Support Foundation http://www.msnews.org/ The Multiple Sclerosis International Federation http://www.ifmss.org.uk/ **Community resources** Have learners visit a trauma or critical care unit to observe types of skeletal trauma. Have learners spend some time with an occupational therapist.

	Journaling How does the client with a spinal cord injury perceive himself or herself? Compare the client's perception with that of people with long-term SCI such as Christopher Reeve. Plan a bladder retraining program for a client with an injury below T-6. **Structured controversy** Too much research money is spent on trying to assist SCI clients to walk again. It should be illegal for lawyers to actively search for and enlist clients with SCI.	

Chapter 44: *Interventions for Clients with Problems of the Peripheral Nervous System*

Learning Outcomes	Learning Activities	Supplemental Resources
After reading this chapter, the student should be able to: 1. Compare and contrast the pathophysiology and etiology of Guillain-Barré syndrome (GBS) and myasthenia gravis. 2. Analyze assessment data for a client with GBS to determine common nursing diagnoses. 3. Prioritize nursing care for the client with GBS. 4. Evaluate nursing care for the client with GBS based on expected outcomes. 5. Identify common clinical manifestations associated with myasthenia gravis (MG). 6. Differentiate between a myasthenic crisis and a cholinergic crisis. 7. Develop a community-based plan of care for the client with MG. 8. Develop a teaching plan for the client with peripheral neuropathy. 9. Prioritize postoperative care for the client undergoing peripheral nerve repair.	**Concept mapping** Have learners map the variations of GBS according to signs and symptoms. Have learners map the pathophysiology of MG with resultant manifestations of signs and symptoms. **Think-pair-share (3-5 min)** What are the most life-threatening complications of Guillain-Barré syndrome? Discuss client education needs for the client with peripheral neuropathy. Why do diabetic clients frequently develop peripheral neuropathy? Discuss the impact of trigeminal neuralgia and facial paralysis on quality of life. What is the role of plasmapheresis in the client with GBS? What is the purpose and implication of electromyography (EMG) testing? What is the relationship between smoking and neuropathy?	Worksheet 44-1 **Internet resources** Guillain-Barré Syndrome Foundation International http://www.webmast.com/gbs/ Guillain-Barré Syndrome Support Group http://www.gbs.org.uk/cidp.html Myasthenia Gravis Foundation of America http://www.myasthenia.org/ Myasthenia Gravis Links for Patients http://pages.prodigy.net/stanley.way/myasthenia/ **Community resources** Have a speech/language and/or occupational therapist demonstrate a speech/swallowing evaluation.

10. Compare and contrast trigeminal neuralgia and radial paralysis. 11. Discuss the role of drug therapy in managing the client with trigeminal neuralgia and facial paralysis. 12. Explain the purpose of surgery for clients with trigeminal neuralgia.	**Journaling** Describe what it must feel like for the client with GBS to be totally cognitively aware but unable to speak. Why would Sleep Pattern Disturbance be an appropriate nursing diagnosis for restless legs syndrome, and what interventions should the nurse plan to implement? **Group learning (15-20 min)** Have groups of learners complete the worksheet on drugs used with myasthenia gravis (MG). In the groups have learners identify the relationship between the drugs and the diagnosis of myasthenic crisis. Learners should be able to discuss the differences between myasthenic crisis and cholinergic crisis. Use Worksheet 44-1. **Campus lab/Clinical component** Have learners develop a plan for communicating with individuals experiencing weakened facial muscles resulting in dysarthric speech.	

Chapter 45: *Interventions for Critically Ill Clients with Neurologic Problems*

Learning Outcomes	Learning Activities	Supplemental Resources
After reading this chapter, the student should be able to: 1. Identify the common types of strokes. 2. Discuss risk factors that increase the likelihood of strokes. 3. Describe typical clinical manifestations associated with stroke. 4. Analyze assessment data to determine common nursing diagnoses that are pertinent to clients with strokes. 5. Identify the purpose of intracranial pressure (ICP) monitoring and signs of increasing ICP. 6. Explain the role of drug therapy in managing clients with strokes. 7. Prioritize nursing care for a client who has experienced a stroke.	**Think-pair-share (3-5 min)** Describe health promotion practices that can decrease the risk of having a stroke. Discuss long-term deficits for clients who sustain severe head injury. What is the difference in the time frame window for the use of thrombolytic therapy in clients with a stroke compared with clients experiencing MI? Identify the major postoperative complications of a craniotomy. Discuss the rationale for the use of different medications for different types of strokes. Why are steroids commonly given to clients with various neurological problems?	**Internet resources** American Brain Tumor Association http://www.abta.org/ National Brain Tumor Foundation http://www.braintumor.org/ The Brain Tumor Society http://www.tbts.org/ National Stroke Association http://www.stroke.org/ National Institute of Neurological Disorders and Stroke http://www.ninds.nih.gov/ **This is a great site for ALL neural disorders.**

8. Discuss the purpose of rehabilitation for the client with a stroke. 9. Develop a teaching plan for the client who has experienced a stroke. 10. Differentiate the common types of traumatic brain injury (TBI). 11. Explain the pathophysiologic changes that can result from moderate or severe TBI. 12. Describe the psychosocial and behavioral manifestations associated with TBI. 13. Prioritize nursing care for the client with TBI. 14. Describe common complications of brain tumors. 15. Develop a postoperative plan of care for a client undergoing a craniotomy.	What is the nurse's role in sending an older adult client back to the nursing home from the emergency department (ED) following evaluation for an apparent head injury? What are the differences and similarities between transient ischemic attacks (TIAs) and reversible ischemic neurologic deficit (RIND)? What are the differences and similarities between shaken baby syndrome and acceleration/deceleration head injuries? What are the differences and similarities between arteriovenous malformation and cerebral aneurysm? Why does an increase in arterial CO_2 exacerbate increased intracranial pressure? What are the rationale, indications, and expected outcomes for the use of mannitol and Decadron in clients with increased intracranial pressure? What is the relationship between amnesia and traumatic brain injury (TBI)? What are the manifestations of Cushings reflex? What is the relationship between increased intracranial pressure and papilledema? What is the rationale for the use of barbiturate-induced coma in clients with elevated ICP? Why might a brain tumor exhibit signs and symptoms earlier than an abdominal tumor? **Concept mapping (10-15 min)** Have learners map the pathophysiology of increasing intracranial pressure (ICP). Have learners map complications of impaired mobility and how to prevent them in clients with neurological disorders. **Pairs check (10-15 min)** Have learners role play having a stroke with right hemiplegia, expressive aphasia, and homonymous hemianopsia. Use eyeglasses on which the same half of each lens is covered with paper. Have learners take turns attempting to ambulate in a wheelchair using only his or her left side. Have learners discuss and practice feeding a client (each other) who has had a CVA; consider placing the food in the appropriate place in the mouth, when to use a syringe, and how to prevent aspiration.	National Aphasia Association http://www.aphasia.org/ The Stroke Network http://www.strokenetwork.org/

	Have learners develop a 2-day diet plan for an individual with impaired swallowing. **Journaling** Prioritize postoperative care for a client having a craniotomy to remove a brain abscess. **Structured controversy (10-15 min)** Should people who do not wear seat belts or safety helmets be cared for using state funds? Is recovery of a severely brain injured client too costly if the victim is over the age of 65? **Numbered heads together (15-20 min)** Assign even-numbered learners to locate data about the cost of disability resulting from strokes. Ask the odd-numbered learners to locate data about the cost of thrombolytic therapy for clients with strokes. Ask a learner from each group to report their findings.	

TM 42-1

NURSING INTERVENTIONS FOR CLIENTS WITH ALZHEIMER'S DISEASE

Stage of Disease	**Appropriate Nursing/ Interdisciplinary Interventions**
Stage I (early)	
Stage II (moderate/middle)	
Stage III (severe/late)	

TM 43-1

COMPARISON OF CHRONIC NEUROLOGICAL DISEASES

	Myasthenia Gravis	Parkinson's Disease	Amyotrophic Lateral Sclerosis	Multiple Sclerosis
Assessment findings				
Cause(s)/risk factors				
Pathophysiology				

TM 44-1

PHARMACOLOGICAL MANAGEMENT OF THE CLIENT WITH MYASTHENIA GRAVIS

Drugs	Mechanism of Action	Anticipated Client Response	Use in Myasthenic Crisis
Anticholinesterases			
Corticosteroids			
Immunosuppressants			

CHAPTER 42

Case Study for the Client with Central Nervous System Disorders

An older client was recently discharged from the hospital for evaluation of seizure activity. His history reveals that he has late-stage Alzheimer's disease, Parkinson's disease, hypertension, and type II diabetes mellitus, which is controlled by diet. He lives at home, where his wife and daughter take care of him. His discharge medications include phenytoin (Dilantin), 100 mg BID; hydrochlorothiazide (HydroDIURIL), 50 mg QD; levodopa (Sinemet), 25/100 TID; and haloperidol (Haldol), 1 mg QN. The client has been referred for home care nursing follow-up.

Questions

1. On the initial home visit by the nurse, what assessments should be made?

2. The wife and daughter need teaching about his antiepileptic medication. What teaching should be included?

3. During the initial home visit, the client experiences a generalized seizure. What action should the nurse take?

CHAPTER 43

Case Study for the Client with a Lumbar Diskectomy

A 35-year-old construction worker was admitted to your unit after an on-the-job accident. He was diagnosed with a herniated nucleus pulposus at L4-5 and had a lumbar diskectomy. This is the client's first hospitalization. He is married and has a 4-year-old daughter, his wife is a school teacher. He has just returned from the PACU.

Questions

1. What is a herniated nucleus pulposus? How would you explain it to the client and his wife?

2. What are your priorities in planning your nursing interventions for this client?

3. How would you get the client out of bed safely?

4. What referrals do you feel are essential for the client in planning his return home?

CHAPTER 44

Case Study for the Client with Guillain-Barré Syndrome

An anxious female client presents in the emergency department (ED) of a community hospital with complaints of leg cramps, lower extremity muscle weakness, and facial weakness. When taking her history, the nurse learns that these symptoms began earlier in the day and have worsened. The client states that she is a physical therapist and is concerned that she may have Guillain-Barré syndrome (GBS). The ED physician confirms this diagnosis and admits the client to the general medical-surgical unit.

Questions

1. What is the nurse's priority in the care of the client at this time?

2. What is a possible cause of the client's GBS?

3. What should the nurse teach her about the disorder?

CHAPTER 45

Case Study for the Client with a Head Injury

A 20-year-old woman fell from a third-story balcony during a fraternity party. Upon arrival, paramedics assessed the following: unresponsive to verbal or painful stimuli, Glasgow Coma Scale score, 3; BP, 70/30; HR, 40 and irregular; R, 6, shallow and irregular; pupils unequal with the right larger than the left and sluggishly responsive; and corneal, cough, and gag reflexes intact. The paramedics resuscitated her in the field and transported her to a regional trauma center on a backboard with a cervical collar in place. She has been intubated and has an orogastric tube and a large-bore IV inserted.

In addition to the neurological injury, the client has a fractured lower leg and an occipital laceration. She has no significant medical history, but her blood alcohol level is 0.17.

In the ED, her status has not changed significantly. Complete laboratory studies, including typing and matching for four units of blood, were done. Extensive x-rays and a CT scan were obtained. The CT scan showed a large left frontoparietal lobe hematoma with a midline shift. The client is taken to the operating room, and a left-sided craniotomy is performed. The epidural hematoma is evacuated, the leg fracture is treated through an open reduction and internal fixation (ORIF), and an intraventricular catheter (IVC) is placed. She is transferred to the ICU.

In the ICU, she received mechanical ventilation and hyperventilated through an endotracheal tube. She has a urinary catheter, an arterial line, and a triple-lumen catheter and is undergoing ECG monitoring and ICP monitoring by means of an IVC. She requires frequent suctioning, turning, and assessment.

Within 3 hours postoperatively, the client is responding appropriately and is able to follow simple commands. Her BP and HR fluctuate but can be controlled with medication. Her ICP ranges between 13 and 25 mm Hg, with the increases noted with nursing activities, and she requires mannitol occasionally for control.

The client's parents have been in to visit and are very upset because she appears to have been drinking at the fraternity party.

Questions

1. What medications can the nurse anticipate the physician ordering for this client?

2. When planning your care for the client, you are aware that many interventions can cause an increase in ICP. How would you plan your nursing care to avoid precipitating an increase in her ICP?

3. What referrals do you think are essential for both the client and her parents in planning for her eventual discharge from the hospital?

4. How would you explain the client's neurological injury to her parents?

UNIT 10 PROBLEMS OF SENSATION: EYES AND EARS ■ Core Concepts Grid

Anatomy	Physiology	Pathophysiology	History	Physical Exam	Diagnostic Tests	Interventions	Pharmacology
• **Cranial nerves** Optic (II) Oculomotor (III) Trochlear (IV) Trigeminal (V) Abducens (VI) Facial (VII) Vestibulo-cochlear (VIII) • **Ears** External canal Tympanic membrane Middle ear Ossicles Eustachian tube Inner ear Semicircular canals Cochlea Endolymph Perilymph Organ of Corti • **Eyes** Eyelids/eyeballs Conjunctiva Lacrimal glands Cornea Uvea Iris/lens/retina Canal of Schlemm Aqueous/vitreous humor	• **Sound transmission** • **Light transmission** • **Color discrimination** • **Refraction** • **Accommoda-tion** • **Coordination**	• **Inflammation** • **Obstruction** • **Tinnitus** • **Vertigo** • **Dizziness** • **Hearing loss** • **Hyperopia** • **Myopia** • **Astigmatism** • **Increased intraocular pressure (IOP)** • **Opacity of lens** • **Retinal detachment** • **Hemorrhage** • **Vision loss**	• **Client past medical history** Systemic medical conditoins Past injuries • **Family history** • **Social history** Medications Occupation Gender Diet history Leisure activities Age	• **Ear** Otoscopic examination Light reflex Voice test Watch test Tuning fork Rinne test Weber test • **Eye** Exophthalmos Ptosis Scleral color Aniscocoria Pupillary reaction Snellen chart Visual fields Jaeger card Six cardinal positions of gaze Corneal light reflex Cover/uncover test	• **Cultures** • **Computed tomography (CT)** • **Audiometry** Bone conduction Pure tone Speech • **Tympanometry** • **Slit-lamp examination** • **Corneal staining** • **Tonometry** • **Ophthal-moscopy** • **Gonioscopy**	• **Ear medication installation** • **Removal of ceru-men** • **Removal of for-eign objects from ear canal** • **Care for the deaf** • **Communication with the deaf** Signing Speech reading • **Eye care** Eye glasses Artificial eyes Contact lenses • **Care for the blind** • **Communication with the blind** Clock TTY Braille	• **Systemic antibi-otics** • **Ear medications** Antibiotic Antifungal Anti-inflammatory • **Antivertigo agents** • **Antiemetics** • **Artificial tears** • **Eye medications** Antibiotic Antifungal Anti-inflammatory • **Midriatics** • **Miotics** Beta blockers Pilocarpine Carbonic anhydrase inhibitors

Unit 10 (Chapters 46-49)

Problems of Sensation: Management of Clients with Problems of the Sensory System

Learning Plan

Chapter 46: *Assessment of the Eye and Vision*

Learning Outcomes	Learning Activities	Supplemental Resources
After reading this chapter, the student should be able to: 1. Explain the concept of refraction in relation to how the cornea, lens, aqueous humor, and vitreous humor contribute to vision. 2. Describe age-related changes in the eye, eyelids, and vision. 3. List five systemic disorders that have an impact on the eye and vision. 4. Discuss which elements of a client's history might predict visual impairment later in life. 5. Discuss the education needs of a client undergoing fluorescein angiography. 6. Explain the relationship between intraocular pressure and eye health. 7. Use proper technique to instill eye drops.	**Think-pair-share (3-5 min)** Describe the anatomy of the eye. Using Worksheet 46-1, ask learners to identify on which areas the nurse should focus and what the nurse should do to perform a physical assessment on this client. Describe eye changes associated with aging. Using Worksheet 46-1, have learners select those data relevant to a subjective assessment and discuss their significance. Why might inquiring about a client's place of employment be applicable to an eye assessment? List at least two reasons why some people prefer contact lenses to eyeglasses. Describe the use of the tonometer. **Pairs check (10-15 min)** Have pairs of learners demonstrate the use of the Snellen chart. Have pairs of learners perform a funduscopic examination. Demonstrate how to manipulate an ophthalmoscope, and discuss the significance of the diopter setting and what to do if the examiner wears corrective lenses. **Campus lab/Clinical component** Demonstrate the appropriate technique for administration of eye drops or ointment. If the situation presents itself, have learners administer eye drops to clients. **Concept mapping (5-10 min)** Map how light is transmitted to the eye.	**Internet resources** All About Vision http://www.allaboutvision.com/resources/anatomy.htm The Vision Correction Website http://www.lasersite.com/ **Community resources** Have learners spend a morning with a local ophthalmologist or optometrist and observe how visual assessments are performed. Have learners research the training and supervising of Seeing Eye dogs.

Chapter 47: *Interventions for Clients with Eye and Vision Problems*

Learning Outcomes	Learning Activities	Supplemental Resources
After reading this chapter, the student should be able to: 1. Describe how to correctly instill ophthalmic drops and ointment into the eye. 2. Explain the consequences of increased intraocular pressure (IOP). 3. Identify common practices that increase IOP. 4. Prioritize educational needs for the client after cataract surgery with and without lens replacement. 5. Compare and contrast myopia and hyperopia and the correction needed for each. 6. Discuss the pathologic bases, symptoms, and nursing care priorities for primary open-angle glaucoma and acute angle-closure glaucoma. 7. Identify the nursing care priorities for the donor when corneal donation is planned. 8. Explain how diabetes mellitus and hypertension affect vision. 9. Prioritize educational needs for the client after corneal transplantation. 10. Describe the common visual deficits for the client with dry macular degeneration. 11. Identify nursing interventions to promote home safety for the client with impaired vision.	**Think-pair-share (3-5 min)** What is hyperemia and keratitis? What are the differences between diplopia as an eye disorder and as a side effect of medications? What effect do diabetes and hypertension have on vision? Why is there a lack of long-term successful outcomes for those clients with long-standing blindness who have their vision surgically restored later in adulthood? What are the systemic effects of glaucoma medications? What are the effects of caffeine on intraocular pressure? What evidence supports a diagnosis of social isolation in a client with vision impairment? Discuss why the diabetic client with retinopathy should stop driving. Discuss why some people "outgrow" their myopia. Discuss the implications of inadequate vitamin A intake on night vision. What adaptations can be anticipated in clients with decreased vision? What is the role of antioxidant vitamins in the prevention of cataracts? What implications does the Americans with Disabilities Act (ADA) have for health care providers? For health care regulatory agencies? Describe the care of the client with contact lenses. Explain how to tell a blind client the location of items in a room or on the food tray. Discuss the use of sunglasses in the prevention of cataracts. Why should farmers, postal workers, and other outdoor workers routinely use sunglasses with ultraviolet ray protection? **Journaling** Which is more difficult: to never have had vision or to lose vision during early childhood? Assign learners to explore the availability of community resources and support groups for blind people.	Worksheet 47-1 **Internet resources** American Foundation for the Blind http://www.afb.org/ Eye Bank Association of America http://restoresight.org/ Blindness Resource Center http://www.nyise.org/blindness.htm The Seeing Eye http://www.seeingeye.org/ Glaucoma Foundation http://www.glaucoma-foundation.org/index.htm The Glaucoma Research Foundation http://www.glaucoma.org/ The National Eye Institute http://www.nei.nih.gov/publications/cataracts.htm American Society of Cataract and Refractive Surgery http://www.ascrs.org/eye/eye.html Antioxidants http://www.antiox.com/findex.html **Community resources** Have groups of learners visit an outpatient surgery unit to observe preoperative and postoperative teaching and care for the client undergoing cataract surgery.

Pairs check (10-15 min)

Ask learners to complete Worksheet 47-1 prior to class. In class ask learners to identify why various classes of medications are used and what outcomes would indicate that the medications were not doing what they were intended to do.

Campus lab/Clinical component

Assign learners to a partner and have each spend 1 hour or more with their eyes covered with eye patches. Have them walk around with the assistance of the other and feed one another.

Practice describing the location of food items on a tray and have the other learner eat according to those directions.

Give each learner a paper grid or graph paper plus a set of three shapes (square, triangle, rectangle). Have learners sit back-to-back. Ask one learner to place the objects on his or her grid and then describe for his or her partner where the partner is to place the matching set of objects on the grid. Allow each to look at the final project. Have learners talk about their experiences in class.

Concept mapping (15-20 min)

Ask learners to map the nursing care of a client who has undergone an abrupt loss of vision.

Ask learners to map the nursing care of a client with glaucoma.

Structured controversy (10-15 min)

Driver's licenses should be revoked for people older than 74.

Insurance companies should be required to pay for clients to have nearsightedness corrected by means of surgery instead of by eyeglasses or contact lenses.

An employer must be able to restrict the hiring of visually impaired individuals.

Chapter 48: *Assessment of the Ear and Hearing*

Learning Outcomes	Learning Activities	Supplemental Resources
After reading this chapter, the student should be able to: 1. Describe the key elements to inspect when performing assessment of the external ear. 2. Describe age-related changes in the structure of the ear and hearing. 3. Identify 10 drugs that have an impact on hearing. 4. Demonstrate the correct use of an otoscope. 5. Describe the landmarks of the tympanic membrane. 6. Compare and contrast air conduction and bone conduction of sound. 7. Demonstrate the correct use of a tuning fork in performing the Weber and Rinne tests for hearing. 8. Prioritize educational needs for the client about to undergo pure tone audiometry and electronystagmography.	**Think-pair-share (3-5 min)** Identify ear changes associated with aging. Contrast sensory and conduction deafness. What hearing changes occur from occupational and recreational activities (when 80 decibels or more are encountered over extended periods)? What evidence supports a diagnosis of social isolation in a client with hearing impairment? Discuss the effects of ototoxic drugs on hearing. What is the purpose of the Rinne and Weber tuning fork test? What is the nurse's responsibility for electronystagmography? What is the function of the bone in hearing? Why is irrigation not used during removal of a foreign body from the ear? What are the symptoms of a perforated eardrum? What factors or conditions can lead to the development of tinnitus? Why can vertigo precipitate nausea? Identify individuals most at risk for developing Meniere's disease. What drugs are effective in the management of Meniere's disease? What are the most common causes of hearing loss? How does a cochlear implant assist with the restoration of hearing? **Journaling** Have learners explore the availability of community resources for hearing impaired individuals. Assign learners to visit a workplace that is known to have an abundance of noise and investigate how the employer minimizes hearing loss that could develop. Also have the learners investigate OSHA guidelines.	**Internet resources** American Speech-Language-Hearing Association http://www.asha.org/ Rights of Deaf And Hard of Hearing Under the ADA http://www.zak.co.il/deaf-info/old/ada_rights.html Self Help for Hard of Hearing People http://www.shhh.org/ Antioxidants http://www.antiox.com/findex.html

	Concept mapping (15-20 min) Have learners draw a map demonstrating how hearing occurs. Include the anatomic structures responsible in the map. Have learners draw a map demonstrating the development of otitis media to the perforation of the eardrum. **Campus lab/Clinical component** With a partner demonstrate the appropriate use of an otoscope. Identify how a fluid filled or infected ear would look from the view of an otoscope. Have learners get a "hearing test" and assist with testing during a local health fair.	

Chapter 49: *Interventions for Clients with Ear and Hearing Problems*

Learning Outcomes	Learning Activities	Supplemental Resources
After reading this chapter, the student should be able to: 1. Compare and contrast the clinical manifestation and interventions for external otitis and otitis media. 2. Describe how to correctly instill medications into the ear. 3. Explain the procedures to safely remove impacted cerumen from the ear canal of an older client. 4. Prioritize educational needs for the client with Meniere's disease. 5. Compare and contrast the causes and interventions for conductive versus sensorineural hearing loss. 6. Prioritize nursing care needs for the client after tympanoplasty. 7. Prioritize nursing care needs for the client after stapedectomy.	**Think-pair-share (3-5 min)** Why is boxer's ear often referred to as *cauliflower ear?* Why is external otitis often referred to as *swimmer's ear?* What adaptations can be anticipated in clients with decreased hearing? Describe the maintenance of hearing aids. Describe the hearing achieved with a hearing aid. Identify the types of sounds lost in different hearing conditions and sounds not heard as well by the older adult. **Journaling** Ask learners to investigate the training of hearing ear dogs and how the deaf person becomes accustomed to working with the dog. **Structured controversy (5-10 min)** A deaf person should not be able to obtain a driver's license.	**Internet resources** American Tinnitus Association http://www.ata.org/ Cochlear Implants http://www.cochlearimplant.com/ Communication Disorders Research http://libweb.sdsu.edu/scidiv/ComDis.html Menieres.org http://www.menieres.org/ Meniere's Disease http://www.teleport.com/~veda/menieres.html

8. Identify an appropriate method for communicating with a client who has recently become hearing impaired. 9. Develop a teaching plan for a client who is learning to use a hearing aid.		

WORKSHEET 46-1

Client History—Sensory Assessment

A nurse at the local Senior Center made the following notation about a client: A 74-year-old female client wearing eyeglasses with bifocal lenses and hearing aid in her left ear. Walks with a shuffling gait, using a cane for support. Wearing house slippers and housedress. States, "My other doctor says I should have my eyes looked at by an expert. It's been a while, and my eyes seem to be acting up lately. I can't see so good anymore." The client states that she takes medication for "sugar" and her blood pressure and has worn glasses for years with the last prescription changed about 3 years ago. "I was a seamstress for many years and quit when I couldn't see to thread the needles anymore—just in time too. These new materials are too hard to work with!" Denies using any eye drops. Describes vision changes as difficulty seeing well at night, especially if trying to read. Uses a magnifying glass to help when reading. No eye pain or discharge, although eyes sometimes feel "dry and scratchy," with the left eye being worse than the right. Admits to rubbing eyes but without relief.

TM 47-1

EYE MEDICATIONS

Drug/Dosage	Classification	Desired Effect	Side/Adverse Effects	Nursing Interventions
Cyclopentolate (Cyclogyl)				
Atropine sulfate				
Acetazolamide (Diamox)				
Pilocarpine				
Physiostigmine				
Phenylephrine (Neo-Synephrine)				

CHAPTER 47

Case Study for the Client with Acute Angle-Closure Glaucoma

One of your assistive nursing personnel, a 45-year-old woman, comes to you complaining of sudden, excruciating pain around the left eye and left cheek, accompanied by nausea. She asks if she can lie down for a while. While talking to her you notice that her left pupil is dilated more than the right and does not react when you move the client from a dimly lit room to one that is brighter. You also notice that the sclera of the left eye is red with enlarged blood vessels radiating outward from the iris. She is anxious and crying.

Questions

1. What assessment techniques should you perform?

2. What questions should you ask?

3. Given these findings, what should be your plan of action?

4. What are the expected outcomes for this situation?

CHAPTER 49

Case Study for the Client with External Otitis

A 38-year-old woman comes to your ambulatory care clinic with complaints of left ear pain for the past 3 days and new onset of purulent green-yellow ear drainage. She describes the pain as aching, and a feeling of fullness in her left ear as well. She denies fever, anorexia, fatigue, and malaise. The client states she has a history of recurrent external ear infections.

Questions

1. What else should you ask the client?

2. What physical signs might you expect in a client with external otitis?

3. What teaching would you reinforce to prevent the recurrence of external otitis?

4. What expected outcomes would be specific to this situation?

UNIT 11 PROBLEMS OF MOBILITY: MUSCULOSKELETAL SYSTEM ■ Core Concepts Grid

Anatomy	Physiology	Pathophysiology	History	Physical Exam	Diagnostic Tests	Interventions	Pharmacology
• **Skeletal System** Bones Cartilage Tendons Ligaments Joints • **Muscular system**	• **Calcium storage** • **Hematopoesis** • **Protection** • **Form/framework** • **Motion** • **Joint articulation**	• **Fracture** • **Sprain** • **Contusion** • **Trauma** • **Osteoporosis** • **Infection**	• **Client medical history** Injury Illness Musculoskeletal Systemic • **Family history** Congenital problems • **Social history** Occupation Sports Nutrition Age Race Gender • **Risk factors** Diet Exercise	• **Joint appearance** • **Gait** • **Range of motion** • **Flexion** • **Extension** • **Hyperextension** • **Abduction** • **Adduction** • **Pronation** • **Supination** • **Circumduction** • **Rotation** • **Inversion** • **Eversion** • **Alignment** • **Bruising/skin trauma** • **Kyphosis**	• **Radiologic studies** • **Arthroscopy** • **Magnetic resonance imaging (MRI)** • **Bone scan** • **Serum calcium** • **Serum phosphorus**	• **Cast care** • **Traction** • **Neurovascular checks** • **Braces/splints** • **Pin tract care** • **Skin assessment** • **Positioning** • **Logroll turning** • **Range-of-motion exercises** • **Body alignment** • **Lifestyle modifications** Diet Exercise • **Rest** • **Physical rehabilitiation** • **Preventing immobility complications**	• **Analgesics** • **Muscle relaxants** • **Nonsteroidal anti-inflammatory drugs (NSAIDs)** • **Antibiotics** • **Calcium** • **Vitamin D** • **Selective estrogen receptor modulators** • **Anticoagulants**

Unit 11 (Chapters 50-52)

Problems of Mobility: Management of Clients with Problems of the Musculoskeletal System

Learning Plan

Chapter 50: *Assessment of the Musculoskeletal System*

Learning Outcomes	Learning Activities	Supplemental Resources
After studying this chapter, the student should be able to: 1. Recall the anatomy and physiology of the musculoskeletal system. 2. Perform a musculoskeletal assessment using Gordon's Functional Health Patterns. 3. Evaluate important assessment findings in a client with a musculoskeletal health problem. 4. Explain the use of laboratory testing for a client with a musculoskeletal health problem. 5. Identify the use of radiography in diagnosing musculoskeletal health problems. 6. Plan follow-up care for clients undergoing musculoskeletal diagnostic testing.	**Think-pair-share (3-5 min)** Identify the anatomy of the musculoskeletal system (muscles, bones, and joints). Describe the normal function of the musculoskeletal system. Identify the physiology of skeletal muscle contraction. Describe the assessment of physical, emotional, and sociological changes in clients with musculoskeletal disorders. Describe the effects of immobility on the musculoskeletal system. Discuss how the nurse assumes the role of coach or uses techniques such as positive reinforcement or behavior modification to help the client adapt to changes brought about by musculoskeletal problems. Describe the loss of calcium from bone during periods of immobility (including a review of the endocrine system and specifically the activities of the parathyroid glands). Describe how abuse, trauma, and disease may alter joint function. Identify the essential components and documentation of neurovascular assessments. Contrast giantism and dwarfism. Based on an assessment of physical, emotional, and sociologic changes in a client with a musculoskeletal disorder, identify measurable goals in the care plan. What medications could alter laboratory tests? What family changes may occur (e.g., job satisfaction or returning to work) when a family member has musculoskeletal problems? Identify examples of personal, diet, and socioeconomic effects on musculoskeletal development.	**Internet resources** Encyclopedia.com: Orthopedics – Current articles in the specialty available http://www.encyclopedia.com/articles/09660.html **Community resources** Show an x-ray of a normal bone and a bone with a fracture. Ask a nurse from a pain clinic to discuss the care of clients with chronic back pain.

	Pairs check (10-15 min) Have learners do a history and physical of the orthopedic system on any client and submit it for review. Note passive and active range of motion (ROM) exercises for each joint. Demonstrate the principles of proper body mechanics. **Concept mapping (10-15 min)** Map the musculoskeletal system.	

Chapter 51: *Interventions for Clients with Musculoskeletal Problems*

Learning Outcomes	Learning Activities	Supplemental Resources
After studying this chapter, the student should be able to: 1. Explain the risk factors for primary and secondary osteoporosis. 2. Describe ways to decrease the risk for osteoporosis. 3. Discuss the role of drug therapy in the prevention and management of osteoporosis. 4. Compare and contrast osteoporosis and osteomalacia. 5. Identify common assessment findings in clients with Paget's disease of the bone. 6. Differentiate acute and chronic osteomyelitis. 7. Analyze assessment data to determine common nursing diagnoses and collaborative problems for the client with a malignant bone tumor. 8. Discuss the psychosocial aspects associated with a diagnosis of bone cancer. 9. Develop a community-based plan of care for a client with a malignant bone tumor. 10. Evaluate the nursing care of a client with a bone tumor using expected outcome criteria. 11. Explain the pathophysiology and risk factors for carpal tunnel syndrome.	**Think-pair-share (3-5 min)** Identify how bone is living tissue. Identify the five stages of bone graft incorporation. Explain the epidemiology and risk factors of osteoporosis. How is osteoporosis measured? Plan a diet for a client with osteoporosis. How can bone resorption in bedridden clients be prevented? Why may renal stones be a problem in clients with osteoporosis? Discuss the role of steroids in the development of osteoporosis. What are the dietary risk factors for development of osteoporosis? List the benefits and risks of hormone replacement therapy (HRT) in postmenopausal women. Compare and contrast the various types of calcium replacement agents. Identify data that best indicate the metabolism of calcium and vitamin D. How does nutrition affect the development of osteoporosis (e.g., the client with anorexia nervosa)? Describe the role of exercise in the prevention of osteoporosis.	**Internet resources** Paget Foundation http://www.paget.org/ National Osteoporosis Foundation http://www.nof.org/ International Osteoporosis Foundation http://www.osteofound.org/ Osteoporosis and Women's Health.com http://www.osteoporosis-and-womens-health.com/ Frequently Asked Questions About Bone Cancer http://www.cancerindex.org/ccw/faq/ **Community resources** Show an x-ray of a joint with degenerative changes. Interview an individual who is experiencing a chronic musculoskeletal problem. Document methods used (past and present) to treat the problem. Examine educational material available from the National Osteoporosis Foundation regarding prevention and treatment of the disease.

12. Discuss treatment options for the client diagnosed with carpal tunnel syndrome. 13. Describe common disorders of the foot, including hallux valgus and plantar fasciitis. 14. Explain the role of the nurse when caring for a client with muscular dystrophy.	What is the impact of long-term isolation for clients isolated with osteomyelitis? Explain wound and skin isolation, contact isolation, and drainage precautions. Identify the principles of perioperative nursing management for the client undergoing musculoskeletal surgery. **Concept mapping (10-15 min)** Map the risk factors of elderly women for osteoporosis. Identify related treatment measures. **Pairs check (10-15 min)** Role-play client teaching strategies for musculoskeletal disease, such as how to teach clients upper arm strengthening and quadriceps sitting exercises. Demonstrate transfer techniques from bed to chair, bed to wheelchair, and wheelchair to toilet. Practice using a sliding board to move a client from bed to stretcher and back. Practice making an orthopedic bed for a client who is a total lift and for a client who can assist by using an overbed trapeze.	Have learners visit the x-ray department to observe x-rays, films, MRIs, and CT scans being done. Have them report about how findings are interpreted.

Chapter 52: *Interventions for Clients with Musculoskeletal Trauma*

Learning Outcomes	Learning Activities	Supplemental Resources
After studying this chapter, the student should be able to: 1. Compare and contrast common types of fractures. 2. Discuss the usual healing process for bone. 3. Identify common complications of fractures. 4. Explain the typical clinical manifestations that are seen in clients with one or more fractures. 5. Analyze common nursing diagnoses for the client with a fracture. 6. Describe the nursing care of the client with a cast, including client education.	**Algorithm** Have learners complete TM 52-1 prior to coming to class. Ask even-numbered learners to develop a decision tree for selecting the type of traction and the type of fracture. Ask odd-numbered learners to develop a decision tree for determining the critical nursing interventions that must accompany the type of traction. **Think-pair-share (3-5 min)** Identify the principles of hot and cold therapies and when each should be used with strains and sprains as result of injuries.	**Transparency master** TM 52-1 Comparison of traction **Internet resources** American Association of Occupational Health Nurses http://www.aaohn.org CDC: Falls and Hip Fractures Among Older Adults http://www.cdc.gov/ncipc/factsheets/falls.htm KidsHealth: The Facts About Fractures and Broken Bones http://kidshealth.org/kid/ill_injure/aches/broken_bones.html

<table>
<tr>
<td>7. Describe the nursing care of the client in traction.
8. Discuss pain management for the client with a fracture.
9. Prioritize nursing care for the postoperative client who has undergone open reduction with internal fixation of the hip.
10. Evaluate the nursing care of a client with a fracture.
11. Identify common types of amputations.
12. Explain the psychosocial aspects related to amputations.
13. Develop a community-based teaching plan for a client who has undergone an elective amputation.
14. Describe the collaborative management for the client with complex regional pain syndrome.
15. Identify the common types of sports-related injuries and their management.</td>
<td>Describe the nurse's role in providing cast care.
What is the significance of epiphyseal plate fractures?
Describe the pathogenesis of fat embolism.
Describe compartment syndrome.
Explain how orthostasis is minimized each time a client is moved to an upright position. What is the rationale for using a tilt table for a client who has been bedridden for a long time?
Compare limb amputation with mastectomy.
Identify the steps the client goes through to eventually accept an amputation.
Describe the "coning" process to shape the residual limb for fit with a prosthetic device.
Describe activities the client is taught to toughen the limb in preparation for a prosthetic device.
Identify the changes a client experiences in adapting to prosthesis.
Describe the body image changes that occur with physically altering surgery.
Identify the types of overuse injuries seen in baseball players, football players, basketball players, tennis players, ballet dancers, runners, cyclists, horseback riders, golfers, data processors, and professional seamstresses.
Discuss the salaries of professional athletes. Does the money offset the cost of treating the physical injuries that will plague them in later years?
What is the nurse's role in sending a client home from the ED with a wet cast on a fresh injury?
What are the possible benefits and risks of NSAIDs and corticosteroids to decrease inflammation before and after arthroscopy?
Why is SQ heparin used prophylactically in clients with orthopedic problems leading to decreased mobility?</td>
<td>Amputation Prevention Global Resource Center
http://www.diabetesresource.com/

Amputee Coalition of America
http://www.amputee-coalition.org/

The Virtual Sports Injury Clinic
http://www.sportsinjuryclinic.net/

Community resources
Have learners accompany a physical therapist and observe gait training and equipment.

Apply an arm cast to learners during one clinical day and remove it 2 days later. Use caution not to cast the elbow or wrist. Have learners report the feelings of being casted (e.g., itching, warmth, lack of motion, and heaviness).

Visit a sports medicine clinic and have a physician describe this specialty and how treatment is provided, with special emphasis on follow-up care.

Ask an orthopedic technician to describe and demonstrate traction devices.

Ask an orthopedic technician to describe the various types of cast materials available—including lightweight and waterproof types.</td>
</tr>
</table>

Pairs check (10-15 min)
Practice using crutches, a cane, and a walker.
Have learners apply elastic bandages and antiembolic hose to each other.
Apply skin traction to one learner and have the other learners practice turning the client, making the bed, and placing the client on a bedpan.
Describe or demonstrate skeletal traction pin site care.

Concept mapping (10-15 min)
Map the different types of limb amputations and their indications and nursing care postoperatively.
Map phantom limb pain and identify methods to treat it effectively.

Numbered heads together (15 min)
Assign even-numbered learners to locate data on the cost of treating a variety of sports-related injuries, including lost wages, pain medications, and pain therapy. If possible, the data should indicate the effects of the injuries on the client 20 to 30 years after the injury.
Ask odd-numbered learners to locate data on the costs of traditional knee surgery versus arthroscopic knee surgery. If possible, the data should indicate the cost of the surgery, hospitalization, and time away from work. Ask a learner to record a central list of costs for treating sports-related injuries and a learner to record a central list of costs for traditional versus arthroscopic knee surgery. Learners should make certain that their information is valid and report their findings to the entire group.

Journaling (15-30 min)
Ask learners to interview an athlete who has suffered a sports injury to determine the feelings of the athlete about the restrictions imposed by the treatment for the injury. Ask learners to pay particular attention to any development issues that surface.
What is the nurse's role in performing a screening health assessment and physical examination for children who go out for team sports?

	Structured controversy (10-15 min) Anabolic steroids, DMSO, and the freezing or numbing of body parts injured in sports should not be used so that the injured person can be allowed to return to play.	

TM 52-1

COMPARISON OF TRACTION

Type	Indication	Length of Procedure	Equipment	Nursing Considerations
Manual				
Skin				
Skeletal				

CHAPTER 51

Case Study for the Client with Acute Osteomyelitis

A 58-year-old man with a foot wound and a history of diabetes mellitus, coronary artery disease hypertension, and pulmonary emphysema sees his nurse practioner. He states that he attempted to cut out an ingrown toenail last week, but his "little knife" slipped and entered the soft tissue around the nail. On inspection, the area is red, warm, and slightly tender. He has a temperature of 101.8° F (39° C).

Questions

1. What other physical assessment should be performed at this time?

2. What laboratory tests will the nurse practitioner most likely order?

3. What treatments may the client have based on his probable diagnosis?

CHAPTER 52

Case Study for the Client with a Fractured Hip

An elderly resident in a nursing home falls during a dance activity in the dayroom. When you check her, you find that she is grimacing and complains of severe left knee pain. Her left leg is slightly externally rotated, and you suspect a fractured hip. She cries and tells you that she is afraid that she has a fractured hip and will die like her best friend did last year.

Questions

1. What other assessments should you conduct at this time?

2. What should you tell the resident to allay her fears?

3. What will the most likely treatment be for the resident after she is admitted to the hospital?

Problems of Digestion, Nutrition, and Elimination: GI System ■ Core Concepts Grid

Anatomy	Physiology	Pathophysiology	History	Physical Exam	Diagnostic Tests	Interventions	Pharmacology
• **Oropharynx** • **Esophagus** • **Stomach** • **Small intestine** • **Large intestine** • **Liver** • **Gallbladder** • **Pancreas** • **Rectum** • **Anus**	• **Absorption** • **Specialized secretions** • **Digestion** Hydrochloric acid Lipase Amylase • **Phagocytosis** • **Coagulation** • **Synthesis of** Proteins Carbohydrates Fat Vitamins • **Detoxification**	• **Inflammation** • **Infection** • **Obstruction** • **Hemorrhage** • **Perforation** • **Dumping syndrome** • **Erosion** • **Ascites**	• **Client history of** Past problems Pain • **Family history of digestive system problems** • **Social history** Alcohol Drugs Stress management Occupation Age Race Gender • **Bowel habits** • **Diet**	• **Mouth** • Skin Striae Cullen's sign Grey-Turner's sign Color • **Peristalsis** • **Bowel sounds** • **Bruits** • **Tympany** • **Masses** • **Abdominal distention** • **Swallowing** • **Intake** • **Vital signs**	• **Upper/lower GI series** • **Endoscopy** • **Esophagastroduodenoscopy (EGD)** • **Endoscopic retrograde cholangiopancreatography (ERCP)** • **Ultrasonography** • **CAT scan** • **Liver biopsy** • **Gastric analysis** • **Fecal analysis** • **Serum bilirubin** • **Aspartate aminotransferase (AST)** • **Alanine aminotransferase (ALT)** • **Lactate dehydrogenase (LDH)** • **Amylase** • **Lipase** • **Culture *Helicobacter pylori***	• **Therapeutic diets** • **Saline lavage** • **Sclerotherapy** • **Tamponade** • **Extracorporeal shock wave lithotripsy (ESWL)** • **Rest** • **Tube** Blakemore Nasogastric Nasoenteric Gastrostomy • **Ostomies** Colostomy Ileostomy • **Postoperative care** • **Rest** • **Fluid replacement** • **Blood transfusion** • **Health teaching**	• **Antacids** • **Histamine blockers** • **Vasocontrictors** • **Corticosteroids** • **Anticholinergics** • **Chenodeoxycholic acid** • **Urodeoxycholic acid** • **Immune serum globulin** • **Hepatitis A vaccine (HAV)** • **Hepatitis B vaccine (HBV)** • **Bowel stimulants** • **Antidiarrheals** • **Antibiotics** • **Lactulose** • **Chemotherapeutic agents**

Unit 12 (Chapters 53-61)

Problems of Digestion, Nutrition, and Elimination: Management of Clients with Problems of the Gastrointestinal System

Learning Plan

Chapter 53: *Assessment of the Gastrointestinal System*

Learning Outcomes	Learning Activities	Supplemental Resources
After studying this chapter, the student should be able to: 1. Recall the anatomy and physiology of the gastrointestinal (GI) system. 2. Perform a GI assessment using Gordon's Functional Health Patterns. 3. Evaluate important assessment findings in a client with a GI health problem. 4. Explain the use of laboratory testing for a client with a GI health problem. 5. Identify the use of radiography in diagnosing GI health problems. 6. Plan follow-up care for clients having endoscopic procedures.	**Think-pair-share (3-5 min)** Have learners complete TM 53-1 prior to class. Compare answers. What enzymes or other substances are necessary for the digestion of carbohydrates, fats, and proteins? Where do these substances originate? Name six major functions of the liver. How does diet impact the incidence of GI cancers? Identify the most common clinical manifestations of GI disorders (e.g., anorexia). How can a skin assessment aid in the diagnosis of GI disorders? How do these skin assessment findings vary in dark skinned clients? Identify the essential elements of documenting an abdominal and nutritional assessment. Which radiographic GI procedures require a "bowel prep"? **Pairs check (15-20 min)** Have learners conduct a GI history, including diet history, on any client and submit for review. Have learners perform an abdominal assessment on any client and submit for review. **Concept mapping (10-15 min)** Identify the normal physiologic changes in the GI system associated with aging that can affect drug absorption, metabolism, distribution, and excretion.	**Transparency master** TM 53-1 Common drugs used for GI disorders **Internet resources** American Cancer Society http://www.cancer.org/ Canadian Cancer Society http://www.cancer.ca/ Gastrointestinal Disorders http://www.merck.com/pubs/mmanual/section3/sec3.htm UNC Center for Functional GI & Motility Disorders http://www.med.unc.edu/medicine/fgidc/ Gastrointestinal.net http://www.gastrointestinal.net/ **Community resources** Invite a dietitian to discuss how to calculate a client's nutritional needs, how to determine enteral formulas, and how to evaluate outcomes of nutritional management. Visit an outpatient Radiology Center to observe a client having a radiographic study of the GI tract (e.g., upper GI series, barium enema). Observe a client undergoing an esophogastroduodenoscopy (EGD), endoscopic retrograde cholangiopancreatography (ERCP), or colonoscopy.

Chapter 54: *Interventions for Clients with Oral Cavity Problems*

Learning Outcomes	Learning Activities	Supplemental Resources
After studying this chapter, the student should be able to: 1. Develop a teaching plan for clients who have stomatitis. 2. Explain the common causes of malignant oral tumors. 3. Identify common nursing diagnoses for clients with oral cancer. 4. Prioritize postoperative care for clients undergoing surgery for oral cancer. 5. Develop a teaching plan for community-based care of clients with oral cancer.	**Think-pair-share (3-5 min)** Prepare a teaching plan for the client with stomatitis. Discuss priorities when caring for a client immediately following oral surgery for cancer. Why should wire cutters be kept at the bedside of the client who has a wired jaw? **Concept mapping (10-15 min)** Diagram the alimentary canal from the mouth to the cardiac sphincter—showing the structures and where disorders are most likely to occur.	**Internet resources** The Apthous Stomatitis Web Site http://www.users.qwest.net/~dallas7/aphthous.html HealthlinkUSA: Oral Cancer http://www.healthlinkusa.com/Oral Cancer.htm Cancernet: Oral Cancer http://cancernet.nci.nih.gov/wyntk pubs/oral.htm Oral Cancer Self Examination http://www.umanitoba.ca/outreach/wisdomtooth/exam.htm **Community resources** Invite an oral surgeon to discuss oral cancer prevention and risk factors. Obtain information about smoking cessation courses available to the community. Have a representative visit. Invite an oral cancer survivor who is maintained through either G-tube feedings or TPN to speak about adjustments to his or her lifestyle.

Chapter 55: *Interventions for Clients with Esophageal Problems*

Learning Outcomes	Learning Activities	Supplemental Resources
After studying this chapter, the student should be able to: 1. Explain the pathophysiology of gastroesophageal reflux disease (GERD). 2. Assess the client who is experiencing GERD. 3. Plan the nursing care for clients with GERD. 4. Develop a postoperative teaching plan for the client having hiatal hernia repair.	**Think-pair-share (3-5 min)** Have learners complete TM 55-1 prior to class. Compare answers. Identify the postoperative complications for a client undergoing an esophagogastrostomy. What teaching is needed for the client with a newly diagnosed hiatal hernia?	**Transparency master** TM 55-1 Comparison of esophageal and gastric disorders **Internet resources** Acid Reflux and Heartburn http://www.diagnosishealth.com/gerd.htm

5. Identify the differences in the incidence of esophageal cancer among cultural groups. 6. Describe the risk factors for esophageal cancer. 7. Analyze assessment data to determine common nursing diagnoses for the client with esophageal cancer. 8. Discuss the priorities for postoperative care of the client undergoing surgery for esophageal cancer. 9. Plan community-based care for clients diagnosed with esophageal cancer.	**Journaling (20-30 min)** Manage care for a client having hiatal hernia repair. Establish realistic outcomes for a client who has had esophageal surgery. Pay particular attention to nutritional needs.	Bedge: A New Way to Cope with Heartburn and Reflux http://bedge.com/ **Community resources** Have learners visit a local drugstore to determine the kinds of antacids and histamind antagonists that are currently available across the counter; note the electrolyte content in each antacid. Invite a radiologist to show x-rays of clients with GERD.

Chapter 56: ***Interventions for Clients with Stomach Disorders***

Learning Outcomes	Learning Activities	Supplemental Resources
After studying this chapter, the student should be able to: 1. Compare etiologies and assessment findings of acute and chronic gastritis. 2. Describe the key components of collaborative management for clients with gastritis. 3. Compare and contrast assessment findings associated with gastric and duodenal ulcers. 4. Identify the most common medical complications that can result from peptic ulcer disease (PUD). 5. Analyze assessment data to determine common nursing diagnoses associated with PUD. 6. Develop a teaching plan related to drug therapy for clients experiencing PUD. 7. Prioritize interventions for clients with upper gastrointestinal bleeding. 8. Plan preoperative and postoperative care for the client undergoing gastric surgery. 9. Develop a community-based plan of care for clients who have undergone gastric surgery. 10. Evaluate outcomes for clients with PUD. 11. Explain Zollinger-Ellison syndrome and its associated clinical manifestations.	**Think-pair-share (3-5 min)** Prepare a client teaching plan to prevent dumping syndrome for clients who have gastric surgery. Prepare a diet-teaching plan for the client with PUD or gastritis. Why is conscious sedation typically used for clients having endoscopic procedures (e.g., EGD or colonoscopy). Why are gastric secretion specimens analyzed? **Journaling (10 min)** Have learners record their observations of clients having diagnostic procedures. Focus on the psychosocial aspects and posttest care.	**Internet resources** Peptic Ulcer Disease http://www.diagnosishealth.com/ulcer.htm Digestive Diseases http://www.niddk.nih.gov/health/digest/digest.htm Zollinger-Ellison Syndrome http://www.niddk.nih.gov/health/digest/summary/zolling/zolling.htm **Community resources** Invite a Radiology/Special Procedures nurse to discuss GI diagnostic tests, including pretest and posttest care. View GI x-rays of clients with intestinal obstruction. Invite a nurse who works in a GI diagnostic clinic to discuss endoscopic procedures, including pretest and posttest care.

12. Analyze risk factors for gastric carcinoma, including cultural considerations. 13. Plan postoperative care for clients who have undergone surgery for gastric cancer. 14. Discuss the psychologic and emotional concerns of clients with gastric cancer.		

Chapter 57: *Interventions for Clients with Noninflammatory Intestinal Disorders*

Learning Outcomes	Learning Activities	Supplemental Resources
After studying this chapter, the student should be able to: 1. Explain the risk factors for irritable bowel syndrome (IBS) and cancer of the colon. 2. Develop a teaching-learning plan for clients with IBS. 3. Differentiate the most common types of hernias. 4. Develop a plan of care for a client undergoing a hernia repair. 5. Interpret diagnostic assessments for clients with colon cancer. 6. Discuss the psychosocial aspects associated with colon cancer and related surgeries. 7. Explain the role of the nurse in managing the client who has colon cancer. 8. Develop a perioperative plan of care for a client undergoing a colon resection and colostomy. 9. Construct a community-based teaching-learning plan for clients requiring colostomy care. 10. Identify community-based resources for clients with colon cancer. 11. Analyze the differences between small-bowel and large-bowel obstructions. 12. Describe assessment findings associated with mechanical and nonmechanical obstructions. 13. Explain the role of the nurse when caring for clients with nasogastric tubes.	**Think-pair-share (3-5 min)** Have learners complete TM 57-1 prior to class. Compare answers. What nursing interventions help prevent aspiration during enteral feedings? Which is more life threatening—small or large bowel obstruction? Why? Identify ways to prevent constipation or diarrhea. Compare and contrast the cost of enteral and parenteral nutrition. **Pairs check (15-20 min)** What are the advantages and disadvantages of large bore nasogastric, small bore nasoduodenal, and gastrostomy tubes for enteral nutrition? Have learners practice inserting nasoenteral tubes on a mannequin/model. Have learners practice checking and documenting placement of nasoenteral tubes on any client using the pH and auscultatory methods. Have learners demonstrate tube feeding using a pump and bolus feeding methods. Have learners demonstrate how to apply a one-and-two piece ostomy system using a model with a stoma. **Concept mapping (15-20 min)** Divide the class into groups of four or five and have them map common concepts for acute versus chronic inflammatory bowel disorders.	**Transparency master** TM 57-1 Comparison of colostomy and ileostomy care **Internet resources** Irritable Bowel Syndrome http://www.gastro.org/public/ibs.html Irritable Bowel/Crohn's Disease http://ibscrohns.about.com/ Cancerlinks http://www.cancerlinks.org/colon.html CancerNet: Colon and Rectal Cancer http://cancernet.nci.nih.gov/Cancer_Types/Colon_And_Rectal_Cancer.shtml **Community resources** Follow a client from the preoperative phase into the operating suite for gastric or intestinal surgery; assist in caring for the client in the PACU. Invite a member of an "ostomy" support group to discuss adaptations with learners.

14. Develop a plan of care for a client experiencing intestinal obstruction. 15. Prioritize nursing care for the client with abdominal trauma.	**Algorithm (10-15 min)** Have learners complete TM 57-1 prior to class, then pair and develop an algorithm for complications associated with colostomy and ileostomy and how to manage them. **Clinical correlation mapping (20-30 min)** Have learners map care for an elderly client who had a bowel resection and transverse colostomy for rectal cancer; the client also has two draining abdominal fistulas.	

Chapter 58: *Interventions for Clients with Inflammatory Intestinal Disorders*

Learning Outcomes	Learning Activities	Supplemental Resources
After studying this chapter, the student should be able to: 1. Compare and contrast the typical physical assessment findings associated with appendicitis and peritonitis. 2. Prioritize nursing care for the client who has peritonitis. 3. Discuss the common causes of gastroenteritis. 4. Compare and contrast the pathophysiology and clinical manifestations of ulcerative colitis and Crohn's disease. 5. Analyze priority nursing diagnoses and collaborative problems for clients with chronic inflammatory bowel disease (IBD). 6. Explain the purpose of and nursing implications related to drug therapy for clients with IBD. 7. Formulate a postoperative plan of care for a client undergoing a colon resection/colectomy and colostomy or ileostomy. 8. Develop a teaching plan for a client needing community-based care for a new ostomy. 9. Identify expected outcomes for clients with chronic IBD.	**Think-pair-share (3-5 min)** Have learners complete TM 58-1 prior to class. Compare answers. Discuss the quality of life for clients with chronic inflammatory disease before and after bowel resection/ostomy. Prepare a teaching plan for a client with diverticular disease. **Numbered heads together (5-10 min)** What are the priority needs of a client who is going home with a new ileostomy (consider physical, psychologic, and social needs)? **Concept mapping (20-30 min)** Have learners develop a plan of care for the client with long-term Crohn's disease. Have learners develop a plan of care for the client with peritonitis following abdominal surgery. Have learners develop a plan of care addressing psychological needs for a woman whose bowel perforated during surgery resulting in an unexpected temporary colostomy.	**Transparency master** TM 58-1 Comparison of common GI inflammatory disorders **Internet resources** Crohn's and Colitis Foundation of America www.ccfa.org/ United Ostomy Association of Canada, Inc. http://www3.ns.sympatico.ca/canada.ostomy/ Ostomies and Stomal Therapy http://www.fascrs.org/coresubjects/ostomies stomal therapy.html **Community resources** Invite an ostomate to discuss lifestyle changes for clients with a colostomy or ileostomy. Invite an enterostomal therapy (ET) nurse to discuss care for clients with ostomies, fissures, and fistulas; also discuss how stoma placement is determined. Have learners participate in rounds with the ET nurse in a hospital or health care setting to assist in ostomy teaching and care.

10. Explain the role of diet therapy in managing the client with diverticular disease. 11. Describe the comfort measures that the nurse can use for the client with an anal abscess, fissure, or fistula. 12. Discuss ways that helminthic infestation, parasitic infection, and food poisoning can be prevented.	**Journaling (20-30 min)** Manage a client postoperatively who has had a bowel resection and descending colostomy. Teach a client being discharged from the hospital and caregivers about ileostomy care. Provide holistic care for a client with long-term Crohn's disease.	Invite a dietitian to describe special diets for clients with GI disorders, including ostomy diets. Invite a vendor (Hollister or Convatec) to demonstrate various products—advantages and disadvantages. (These companies also supply patient education literature, professional education literature and audiovisual aids, and models with stomas for learner practice.) Have learners visit the local health department to obtain information regarding sanitary food practices that must be followed by public restaurants (or contact through e-mail, letter, phone, or Web site).

Chapter 59: *Interventions for Clients with Liver Problems*

Learning Outcomes	Learning Activities	Supplemental Resources
After studying this chapter, the student should be able to: 1. Describe the pathophysiology and complications associated with cirrhosis of the liver. 2. Interpret laboratory test findings commonly seen in clients with cirrhosis. 3. Analyze assessment data from clients with cirrhosis to determine priority nursing diagnoses and collaborative problems. 4. Formulate a collaborative plan of care for the client with severe late-stage cirrhosis. 5. Identify emergency interventions for the client with bleeding esophageal varices. 6. Evaluate care for clients with cirrhosis. 7. Develop a community-based teaching plan for the client with cirrhosis of the liver. 8. Compare and contrast the transmission of hepatitis A, B, and C viral infections.	**Think-pair-share (3-5 min)** Discuss the priority in caring for the client immediately following a liver biopsy. What is obstructive jaundice and how does it occur? Describe the relationship of serum ammonia levels and mental status. How are hepatitis A, B, and C similar? How do they differ? Identify the laboratory tests that typically have abnormal results when a client has advanced cirrhosis. Plan a meal for a client with late stage cirrhosis. Describe the quality of life for clients with liver transplants. **Structured controversy (20-30 min)** Should the client with alcoholic cirrhosis be a candidate for a liver transplant? Should government funds be used in the care of clients with cirrhosis who continue to consume alcohol?	**Internet resources** American Liver Foundation http://www.liverfoundation.org/ American Council on Alcoholism http://www.aca-usa.org/ NIDDK: Cirrhosis of the Liver http://www.niddk.nih.gov/health/digest/pubs/cirrhosi/cirrhosi.htm NIDDK: Chronic Hepatitis C – Current Disease Management http://www.niddk.nih.gov/health/digest/pubs/chrnhepc/chrnhepc.htm Hepatitis Foundation Newsletter http://www.hepfi.org/

9. Explain ways in which each type of hepatitis can be prevented. 10. Discuss the primary concerns about the increasing incidence of hepatitis C in the United States. 11. Identify treatment options for clients with cancer of the liver. 12. Describe the typical complications that result from liver transplantation.	**Concept mapping (10-15 min)** Have learners map the pathophysiology of ascites. **Clinical correlation mapping (20-30 min)** Have learners map care for a middle-aged client who has a new liver transplant as a result of chronic hepatitis. **Journaling (20-30 min)** Plan care for a client undergoing a liver transplant across the continuum of care (hospital to home).	CDC: Viral Hepatitis http://www.cdc.gov/ncidod/diseases/hepatitis/ **Community resources** Visit a meeting of Alcoholics Anonymous, Al-Anon, or other support group for families of alcoholics. Invite an Infection Control Nurse to discuss types of hepatitis, prevention, and isolation precautions. Observe management of bleeding esophageal varices in the ED or Critical Care Unit. Observe a liver transplant operation.

Chapter 60: *Interventions for Clients with Problems of the Gallbladder and Pancreas*

Learning Outcomes	Learning Activities	Supplemental Resources
After studying this chapter, the student should be able to: 1. Identify the common causes of cholecystitis and cholelithiasis (gallbladder disease). 2. Explain the role of testing in diagnosis of gallbladder disease. 3. Compare postoperative care of clients undergoing a traditional cholecystectomy with that of clients undergoing a laparoscopic cholecystectomy. 4. Develop a community-based teaching plan for clients with gallbladder disease, including care of a T tube. 5. Compare and contrast the pathophysiology of acute and chronic pancreatitis. 6. Interpret common assessment findings associated with acute pancreatitis and those associated with chronic pancreatitis. 7. Prioritize nursing care for clients with acute pancreatitis and clients with chronic pancreatitis.	**Think-pair-share (3-5 min)** What is the advantage of gallbladder ultrasound over radiographic gallbladder procedures? Describe the clinical manifestations associated with cholelithiasis. Describe the characteristics of pain experienced by clients with acute and chronic pancreatitis. Identify the laboratory tests that typically have abnormal results when a client has acute pancreatitis. What teaching is required for a client being discharged from the hospital with a T tube? **Clinical correlation mapping (20-30 min)** Have learners map care for a young alcoholic client who has acute pancreatitis; have learners share their map with their partners. **Journaling (20-30 min)** Provide collaborative care for a client with acute pancreatitis resulting from alcoholism. Manage care for a client who underwent a traditional cholecystectomy and in whom a T-tube was inserted.	**Internet resources** Laparoscopic gallbladder surgery http://vava.essortment.com/laparoscopicgal_riwj.htm MediLinks: Gall Bladder Disease: Gallstones http://www.yarmouth.org/ps/links/g/gbladder/ The American Gastroenterological Association—Pancreatitis http://www.gastro.org/public/pancreatitis.html NIDDK: Pancreatitis http://www.niddk.nih.gov/health/digest/pubs/pancreas/pancreas.htm The Johns Hopkins Medical Institutions: Pancreas Cancer Home Page http://www.path.jhu.edu/pancreas

8. Explain the use and adverse effects of drug therapy for clients with chronic pancreatitis. 9. Develop a postoperative plan of care for clients undergoing a Whipple procedure. 10. Construct a discharge plan for care of clients with pancreatic cancer in the community. 11. Discuss the psychosocial needs of the client with pancreatic cancer and associated nursing interventions.	Provide collaborative care for a client with pancreatic or liver cancer.	Medical University of South Carolina: Patient Information—Surgeries: Whipple http://www.ddc.musc.edu/ddc pub/patientInfo/surgeries/whipple.htm **Community resources** Observe a pancreatic transplant operation. Follow a client undergoing a laparoscopic cholecystectomy in a same-day surgical setting. Invite a dietitian to discuss the therapeutic diet for a client with gallbladder problems. Interview a Hospice nurse about pain control in the client with terminal pancreatic illness.

Chapter 61: *Interventions for Clients with Malnutrition and Obesity*

Learning Outcomes	Learning Activities	Supplemental Resources
After studying this chapter, the student should be able to: 1. Identify three anthropometric measurements that the nurse can use to evaluate a client's nutritional status. 2. Explain the potential consequences and complications associated with malnutrition. 3. Describe the risk factors for malnutrition, especially for older adults. 4. Discuss the role of laboratory testing in the diagnosis of malnutrition. 5. Analyze assessment data to determine common nursing diagnoses for the client with malnutrition. 6. Identify expected outcomes for clients who are malnourished. 7. Describe the nursing care of clients receiving total enteral nutrition (TEN).	**Think-pair-share (3-5 min)** What are the best indicators (physical and laboratory) for nutritional status? Discuss factors that influence dietary intake in elderly adults. Why do clients receiving TPN require frequent monitoring of weight and blood glucose level? Discuss the effect of morbid obesity on a client's quality of life. Describe interventions to increase food intake for clients with a diminished appetite. **Pairs check (15-20 min)** Have learners conduct a nutritional assessment on any client and submit for review.	**Internet resources** Healthy Weight http://www.healthyweight.com/ NIH News Release: First Federal Obesity Clinical Guidelines Released http://www.nhlbi.nih.gov/new/press/oberel4f.htm TPN pro.com http://www.tnpnutrition.com/ Living Lean Today http://www.livingleantoday.com/ **Community resources** Invite an Office on Aging representative to discuss nutritional programs for the elderly in the community.

<table>
<tr>
<td>8. Prioritize nursing care needs for clients receiving total parenteral nutrition (TPN).
9. Identify complications associated with TPN.
10. Explain the potential consequences and complications associated with obesity.
11. Discuss the role of culture and gender as factors in the prevalence of obesity.
12. Identify the role of drug therapy in the management of obesity.
13. Develop a postoperative teaching plan for clients undergoing a gastroplasty or an intestinal bypass.</td>
<td>Structured controversy (20-30 min)
Should government funds be used for surgical procedures for obese clients who have not been compliant with dietary restrictions?

Journaling (20-30 min)
Have learners care for residents in a nursing home who are being tube fed during their late stage of Alzheimer's disease; have them express their feelings about tube feeding for this type of client, including the cost of the treatment and other family issues.
Provide collaborative care for a client with malnutrition.
Manage a home care client receiving total parenteral nutrition or enteral nutrition.</td>
<td>Have learners participate in rounds with the dietitian to assess clients with tube feedings and parenteral nutrition (TPN).

Make visits with a home health nurse to observe how enteral and parenteral nutrition are provided in the home setting.

Go on a visit with a home care nurse to care for a client with TPN or tube feeding.

Assign learners to provide care for nursing home residents who are being fed through gastrostomy tube.</td>
</tr>
</table>

TM 53-1

COMMON DRUGS USED FOR GASTROINTESTINAL DISORDERS

Drug Classification	Action	Indications for Use	Side/Adverse Effects	Nursing Indications
Antacids (such as Mylanta)				
Histamine antagonists (such as Pepcid)				
Proton pump inhibitors (such as Prilosec)				

TM 55-1

COMPARISON OF ESOPHAGEAL AND GASTRIC DISORDERS

	GERD	PUD	Hiatal Hernia	Gastritis
Pathophysiology				
Etiology				
Clinical manifestations				
Typical nursing diagnoses				

TM 57-1

COMPARISON OF COLOSTOMY AND ILEOSTOMY CARE

	Ascending Colostomy	**Transverse Colostomy**	**Descending/ Sigmoid Colostomy**	**Ileostomy**
Placement of stoma				
Type of effluence (drainage)				
Options for appliance				
Diet considerations				
Management of complications				

TM 58-1

COMPARISON OF COMMON GASTROINTESTINAL INFLAMMATORY DISORDERS

	Gastroenteritis	**Peritonitis**	**Ulcerative Colitis**	**Crohn's Disease**
Pathophysiology				
Etiology				
Clinical manifestations				
Typical nursing diagnoses				

CHAPTER 54

Case Study for the Client with Oral Cavity Cancer

A 56-year-old male client is seen in the clinic and has had a sore in his mouth for 3 months that he claims "isn't healing." He tells you that he is a heavy smoker, but is only a social drinker. He is diagnosed with squamous cell carcinoma. You are meeting with him to review his plan of care.

Questions

1. What lifestyle concerns need to be addressed to plan care?

2. What additional information would be helpful to plan care with this client?

3. This client chooses to have surgical treatment, and a composite resection is scheduled. What instructions should you provide for this client before surgery?

CHAPTER 55

Case Study for the Client with Gastroesophageal Reflux Disease (GERD)

A 59-year-old female client presents in the physician's office with a diagnosis of possible GERD. She has a history of arthritis for which she takes ibuprofen (Motrin) 200 mg QID.

Questions

1. What questions should you ask when taking a history from this woman?

2. What information should you include when making a teaching plan for this client?

CHAPTER 56

Case Study for the Client with Peptic Ulcer Disease (PUD)

A 48-year-old female client comes to the employee health office complaining of heartburn, indigestion, and pain during the night. She is a computer technician and has recently served as the project coordinator at work for an upgrade of computers and software.

She is generally in good health and has no history of health problems or concerns. She does report taking some over-the-counter ibuprofen and antacids as needed, and typically drinks six cups of coffee a day. You ask her to go into the examination room for further assessment.

Questions

1. When taking a complete history from this client, what important questions should you ask?

2. Which components of physical assessment should you perform?

3. She tells you that her stools are dark and appear black. Given this statement, what should you do first?

CHAPTER 57

Case Study for the Client with a Bowel Obstruction

You are making a home visit to a 69-year-old male client who had a stroke when he was aged 59 years. He is wheelchair dependent. Other health concerns include chronic constipation, angina, and social isolation. His only operations were a cholecystectomy and appendectomy at age 45. His only medications are milk of magnesia and nitroglycerin PRN. At the start of the home visit, he tells you, "My bowels have not moved in 1 week; my magnesia is not working."

Questions

1. In this situation, what questions should you ask?

2. Which components of the physical examination should you perform?

3. What health problem(s) may he be experiencing?

4. Which conditions place him at risk for bowel obstruction?

5. During the health assessment, you cannot hear any bowel sounds. His abdomen is distended and tender to touch. On the basis of these assessment findings, what is the most appropriate action?

CHAPTER 58

Case Study for the Client with Inflammatory Bowel Disease

A 68-year-old female client is admitted to the hospital for a colectomy and ileostomy for ulcerative colitis. Her surgeon describes her as extremely anxious. Your client's mother died unexpectedly after surgery about 5 years ago. Her other health problems include hyperthyroidism and anemia. She has had a 30-lb weight loss since the onset of her illness 18 months ago. She has lived alone since her mother's death. She has few friends, and her sisters and brothers visit her infrequently.

Her nasogastric tube is removed 3 days after surgery. The physician has ordered sips of fluids orally. Your client calls you to her room and tells you that her stomach is "going to explode." She appears very restless and is twisting her hands. You begin a further assessment.

Questions

1. Should your assessment initially focus on her physical complaints or her mood and behavior?

2. What further questions should you ask?

3. What are the priority areas of assessment?

4. During the abdominal assessment, you find that her abdomen is distended and there are no bowel sounds. Given these assessment findings, what should you do first?

CHAPTER 59

Case Study for the Client with Cirrhosis

You are a staff nurse on a busy medical unit. One of the nursing assistants tells you that a male client may be confused. You know that your male client, aged 50, was admitted last evening with a medical diagnosis of alcoholic cirrhosis. When you question the nursing assistant about why she feels that he is confused, she responds that he is talking about needing to catch the next bus that goes by his door.

Questions

1. On the basis of the medical diagnosis, what complication may your client be experiencing?

2. What assessment and laboratory data do you need to obtain immediately?

3. What is the usual medical treatment for this complication? Why is this treatment used?

CHAPTER 60

Case Study for the Client with Acute Pancreatitis

You are a charge nurse on a medical unit of a large teaching hosital. The Emergency Department (ED) is sending you a new admission, a female client, age 48, with a medical diagnosis of acute pancreatitis. Upon her arrival to your unit, you fully assess your client. Included in your assessment findings are the following data:

- *VS: T, 100.2° F; P, 104; R, 22; B/P, 100/60*
- *Sharp pain in the midepigastric area radiating to the back, rated as 8 (scale 0-10)*
- *Vomited twice in the ED; reports that she is still nauseated*
- *Bowel sounds hypoactive at 2 per minute*

Questions

1. Why is it important to monitor vital signs of the client with acute pancreatitis?

2. What position may help to decrease the client's pain?

3. What medication will probably be ordered for the client's pain, and why?

4. What do the nausea, vomiting, and hypoactive bowel sounds indicate?

UNIT 13 PROBLEMS OF REGULATION AND METABOLISM: ENDOCRINE SYSTEM ■ Core Concepts Grid

Anatomy	Physiology	Pathophysiology	History	Physical Exam	Diagnostic Tests	Interventions	Pharmacology
• **Glands** Anterior pituitary Posterior pituitary Thyroid Parathyroid Pancreas Adrenal • **Hormones** Antidiuretic hormone (ADH) Thyroid-stimulating hormone (TSH) Adrenocorticotropic hormone (ACTH) Growth hormone (GH) Mineralocorticoids Glucocorticoids Androgens Epinephrine Norepinephrine Thyroxine Thyrocalcitonin Parathormone Insulin Glucagon	• **Neuroregulation** • **Hypothalamus** • **Regulation** Metabolism Fluids/electrolytes Glucose levels Stress response	• **Inflammation** • **Hypersecretion** • **Hyposecretion** • **Infection** • **Diabetic ketoacidosis** • **Hyperglycemic hyperosmolar nonketotic syndrome (HHNKS)** • **Adrenal crisis**	• **Client history** Energy level Elimination pattern Nutrition Reproductive function Libido • **Family history** Endocrine disease • **Social history** Drug/alcohol use Coping skills Age Gender • **Weight change**	• **Appearance** Skin Hair Body fat distribution Muscle mass Bruising Petechiae Edema Face Genitalia • **Size of thyroid** • **Vital signs** • **Weight**	• **Adrenocorticotropic hormone (ACTH) levels** • **Aldosterone assay** • **Antidiuretic hormone (ADH)** • **Blood glucose** • **Catecholamines** Vanillylmandelic acid (VMA) • **Cortisol** • **Glycosolated hemoglobin A_{1c}** • **17-hydroxycorticosteroids** • **Ketones** • **Parathyroid hormone level** • **T_3/T_4** • **Thyroid scan**	• **Hormone replacement** • **Nutrition** • **Fluid management** • **Stress management** • **Client education** Diet Exercise Hormone replacement regimen Overdose Underdose Foot care Signs of complications Need for carrying emergency medical information • **Postoperative care/monitoring for complications** Thyroidectomy Adrenalectomy Pancreas transplantation • **Monitoring for hypoglycemia and hyperglycemia**	• **Glucagon** • **Insulin** • **Oral hypoglycemic agents** • **Thyroid replacement** • **Thyroid inhibitors** • **Pituitary hormone replacements** • **Pituitary hormone inhibitors** • **Parathyroid hormone replacement** • **Parathyroid hormone inhibitors** • **Calcium** • **Adrenal hormone replacements** • **Adrenal hormone inhibitors**

Unit 13 (Chapters 62-65)

Problems of Regulation and Metabolism: Management of Clients with Problems of the Endocrine System

Learning Plan

Chapter 62: *Assessment of the Endocrine System*

Learning Outcomes	Learning Activities	Supplemental Resources
After reading this chapter, the student should be able to: 1. Describe the relationship between hormones and receptor sites. 2. Explain negative feedback as a control mechanism for hormone secretion. 3. Discuss the structure and function of the hypothalamus. 4. Discuss the structure and function of the anterior and posterior lobes of the pituitary gland. 5. Discuss the structure and function of the adrenal glands. 6. Discuss the structure and function of the thyroid and parathyroid glands. 7. Discuss the structure and function of the pancreas. 8. Describe changes in the endocrine system associated with aging. 9. Identify laboratory tests that aid in determining endocrine function and dysfunction.	**Think-pair-share (3-5 min)** What does the term *negative feedback* mean in regard to hormonal functioning? Why is the hypothalamus considered the "master gland"? What is the role of the mineralocorticoids on electrolyte balance? What is the role of the glucocorticoids on glucose levels? What is the relationship between parathyroid functioning and the kidneys? Why is insulin considered an anabolic hormone? What is the effect of aging on the endocrine system? What age-related physical changes in the older adult can lead to misinterpretation of normal laboratory values? **Concept mapping (10-15 min)** Have learners map the relationship among T_3, T_4, and TSH. Ask groups of learners to map connections among the various endocrine glands. Have learners use a body system approach to map the clinical manifestations or bodily appearance changes brought about by disorders of the endocrine system. **Journaling** Consider, from the client's view, the impact of receiving a diagnosis of a disorder in the endocrine system and the wide reaching effect of such a diagnosis on a myriad of body systems.	**Internet resources** The Endocrine System http://encarta.msn.com/find/Concise.asp?ti=05928000

<table>
<tr><th colspan="3">Chapter 63: Interventions for Clients with Pituitary and Adrenal Gland Problems</th></tr>
<tr><th>Learning Outcomes</th><th>Learning Activities</th><th>Supplemental Resources</th></tr>
<tr><td>After reading this chapter, the student should be able to:

1. Compare and contrast the common clinical manifestations associated with pituitary hypofunction and pituitary hyperfunction.
2. Use clinical changes and laboratory data to determine the effectiveness of interventions for pituitary hypofunction.
3. Identify the teaching priorities for the client taking hormone replacement therapy for pituitary hypofunction.
4. Prioritize the nursing care needs of the client immediately after a transsphenoidal hypophysectomy.
5. Use clinical changes and laboratory data to determine the effectiveness of interventions for pituitary hyperfunction.
6. Compare and contrast the problems associated with oversecretion and undersecretion of antidiuretic hormone (ADH).
7. Explain the effect of diabetes insipidus on blood and urine volumes and blood and urine osmolarities.
8. Explain the effect of SIADH on blood and urine volumes and blood and urine osmolarities.
9. Use clinical changes and laboratory data to determine the effectiveness of interventions for diabetes insipidus.
10. Identify teaching priorities for the client with diabetes insipidus.
11. Use clinical changes and laboratory data to determine the effectiveness of interventions for SIADH.
12. Identify teaching priorities for the client with SIADH.
13. Compare and contrast the clinical manifestations of Cushing's syndrome and Addison's disease.</td><td>Think-pair-share (3-5 min)
Compare and contrast giantism and dwarfism.
What is the function of vasopressin?
How might body image be affected by growth hormone and other pituitary hormone abnormalities?
Why are fluids and sodium restricted for the client with Cushing's syndrome?
Why is dehydration a major problem for the client experiencing diabetes insipidus and what nursing interventions should be used to address this problem?
Why is hypernatremia a major problem for the client experiencing SIADH, and what nursing interventions should be used to address this problem?
Why is hyperkalemia a major problem for the client experiencing adrenal hypofunction and what interventions should be used to address this problem?
Why is fluid restriction necessary in the client with SIADH?
Why should a client with Addision's disease or Cushing's syndrome wear a medical alert bracelet?
What is the difference between primary and secondary hyperaldosteronism?
What is the significance of the VMA test in the client with pheochromocytoma?
Why does a pheochromocytoma produce profound hypertension?

Concept mapping (10-15 min)
Have learners map the various hormones secreted by the pituitary gland and their target organs.
Have learners map the pathophysiology of Cushing's syndrome with related clinical manifestations.

Journaling
Discuss how the nurse can assist the client with an altered physical appearance due to hyperpituitarism.
What is the cost of lifelong replacement therapy for Addison's disease?</td><td>Worksheet 63-1

Internet resources
National Adrenal Disease Foundation
http://www.medhelp.org/www/nadf4.htm

Neuroendocrine Clinical Center & Pituitary Tumor Center
http://neurosurgery.mgh.harvard.edu/nendo-hp.htm

Pituitary Network Association
http://www.pituitary.com/

The Addison & Cushing International Federation
http://www.spin.nl/nvap0406.htm</td></tr>
</table>

14. Use clinical changes and laboratory data to determine the effectiveness of interventions for Cushing's syndrome. 15. Identify teaching priorities for the client with Cushing's syndrome. 16. Use clinical changes and laboratory data to determine the effectiveness of interventions for Addision's disease. 17. Identify teaching priorities for the client with Addision's disease.	**Numbered heads together (10-15 min)** Ask learners to complete worksheet 63-1 prior to coming to class. Ask even-numbered learners to identify assessment findings that would indicate excesses and ask odd-numbered learners to identify assessment findings that would indicate deficits. Develop a teaching plan for clients anticipating a transsphenoidal approach to pituitary gland removal.	

Chapter 64: *Interventions for Clients with Problems of the Thyroid and Parathyroid Glands*

Learning Outcomes	Learning Activities	Supplemental Resources
After reading this chapter, the student should be able to: 1. Compare and contrast the common clinical manifestations associated with hyperthyroidism and hypothyroidism. 2. Explain the pathophysiology of Graves' disease. 3. Use clinical changes and laboratory data to determine the effectiveness of interventions for hyperthyroidism. 4. Prioritize the nursing care needs of the client during the first 24 hours following a total thyroidectomy. 5. Explain the pathophysiology of Hashimoto's thyroiditis. 6. Identify teaching priorities for the client taking thyroid hormone replacement therapy. 7. Use clinical changes and laboratory data to determine the effectiveness of interventions for hypothyroidism. 8. Compare and contrast the common clinical manifestations associated with hyperparathyroidism and hypoparathyroidism. 9. Prioritize the nursing care needs of the client during the first 24 hours following a total parathyroidectomy.	**Think-pair-share (3-5 min)** Describe the effects of an increased basal metabolic rate in the client with hyperparathyroidism. Identify why the client with hypoparathyroidism is at risk for tetany and laryngospasm. Why are dairy products restricted in clients with hypoparathyroidism? Explain why parathyroid assessments are necessary for a client following a thyroidectomy. What is the mechanism of action of antithyroid drugs? What is the success of radioactive iodine therapy? Why might the average dose of opioids, barbiturates, and anesthetics be fatal to the client with myxedema? In what situations should the use of iodized salt be encouraged? Why do hypercalcemia clients become toxic from digitalis preparations? What nursing interventions are involved in the client with exophthalmos? What is a goiter, what is its etiology, and how is it related to thyroid disease? What is myxedema coma? How is depression related to hypothyroidism? What is the difference between thyroiditis and thyroid disease? Differentiate between the types of thyroid cancer.	**Internet resources** EndocrineWeb.com http://www.endocrineweb.com/parathyroid.html American Thyroid Association http://www.thyroid.org/ The Thyroid Foundation of America http://www.tsh.org/ Thyroid Federation International http://www.thyroid-fed.org/

10. Use clinical changes and laboratory data to determine the effectiveness of interventions for hyperparathyroidism problems.	**Numbered heads together (10-15 min)** Ask even-numbered learners to explain pharmacological management of clients with hypothyroidism and hyperthyroidism and ask odd-numbered learners to explain pharmacological management of clients with hypoparathyroidism and hyperparathyroidism. Ask even-numbered learners to develop a nursing care plan that includes client teaching about hypo- and hyperthyroidism and ask odd-numbered learners to develop a nursing care plan that includes client teaching about hypo- and hyperparathyroidism. The plans should focus on lifestyle changes that will need to be implemented based on the various diagnoses. Ask even-numbered learners to identify the anesthesia and perioperative management of clients with problems of excess thyroid and parathyroid production. Ask odd-numbered learners to identify the anesthesia and perioperative management of clients with problems of insufficient thyroid and parathyroid production. **Concept mapping (15-20 min)** Have groups of learners map the clinical manifestations of hyperthyroidism compared with hypothyroidism according to body systems. Have learners map the clinical manifestations of thyroid storm and match the manifestations to the anticipated nursing and/or medical interventions involved. **Journaling** What is the cost of lifelong thyroid replacement medications and of thyroid destructive medications such as radioactive iodine? Should clients receiving thyroid replacement use generic or brand name drugs?	

Chapter 65: *Interventions for Clients with Diabetes Mellitus*

Learning Outcomes	Learning Activities	Supplemental Resources
After reading this chapter, the student should be able to: 1. Compare and contrast the age of onset, clinical manifestations, and pathologic mechanisms of type 1 and type 2 diabetes mellitus. 2. Identify clients at risk for developing type 2 diabetes mellitus. 3. Explain the effects of insulin on carbohydrate, protein, and fat metabolism. 4. Evaluate laboratory data to determine whether the client is using the prescribed dietary, medication, and exercise interventions for diabetes. 5. Explain the effect of aerobic exercises on blood glucose levels. 6. Describe the significance of the presence of ketone bodies in the urine of a diabetic client. 7. Use the exchange system to plan a menu for a client with diabetes who is prescribed to eat 1800 calories per day, divided into three meals and a snack, with 15% of calories from fat, 20% of calories from protein, and the remaining calories from carbohydrate sources. 8. Compare the mechanisms of actions of the sulfonylureas, biguanides, alpha-glycosidase inhibitors, and the thiazolidinediones as antidiabetic agents. 9. Explain the effect of hypertension on the development of diabetic nephropathy and diabetic retinopathy. 10. Identify clients at risk for the development of hypoglycemia. 11. Prioritize nursing interventions for the client with mild to moderate hypoglycemia. 12. Prioritize nursing interventions for the client with moderate to severe hypoglycemia. 13. Identify clients at risk for developing diabetic ketoacidosis (DKA).	**Think-pair-share (3-5 min)** Identify the early assessment findings for the diabetic neuropathies. What are the early assessment findings for the diabetic client with nephropathy, neuropathy, and retinopathy? What drugs interfere with oral hypoglycemic agents? Identify the pathophysiological changes related to diabetes. Contrast the differences between the diabetic crises of hypoglycemia and diabetic ketoacidosis. Compare the signs and symptoms of hypoglycemia with acute alcohol intoxication. Identify the pathophysiological changes related to diabetes. Contrast the differences among the diabetic crises of hypoglycemia, diabetic ketoacidosis (DKA), and hyperglycemic hyperosmolar nonketotic coma (HHNC). How might type I diabetes mellitus affect the growth and development of the child and adolescent? What disposal methods for insulin syringes should be used in the home by the diabetic client? What is the general quality of life in clients before and after pancreas, kidney-pancreas, and islet cell transplantation? What are some implications of diabetic clients consuming alcohol as part of the total caloric intake? Discuss cigarette smoking as a modifiable risk factor for NIDDM. What information does a glycosylated hemoglobin level reveal about the compliance of a diabetic client? What are the advantages and disadvantages for the use of implantable pumps, nasal administration, or transdermal administration of insulin? What are the major complications of pancreatic transplantation?	**Internet resources** American Association of Diabetic Educators http://www.aadenet.org/index2.html American Diabetes Association http://www.diabetes.org/ American Dietetic Association http://www.eatright.org/ The Diabetes Monitor http://www.diabetesmonitor.com/ National Institute of Diabetes & Digestive & Kidney Disease http://www.niddk.nih.gov/ **Community resources** Have selected learners spend a day with a diabetic educator. Have selected learners investigate the services of the American Diabetic Association. Have selected learners investigate the location and availability of diabetic support groups.

14. Prioritize nursing interventions for clients with DKA.
15. Identify clients at risk for the developing hyperglycemic hyperosmolar nonketotic syndrome (HHNS or HHNKS).
16. Prioritize nursing interventions for the clients with DKA.
17. Use laboratory data and clinical manifestations to determine the effectiveness of the interventions for DKA and HHNS.
18. Describe the correct technique to use when mixing different types of insulin within the same syringe.
19. Compare and contrast the clinical manifestations of hyperglycemia and hypoglycemia.
20. Perform foot assessment and foot care for the client with diabetes.

Concept mapping (15-20 min)

Ask groups of learners to map what the diabetic client must consider for foreign travel (such as how to obtain insulin or oral hypoglycemic agents and syringes in a foreign country, and taking a Medic Alert bracelet, glucometer glucagon emergency kit, prescription for insulin, and health history).

Have learners develop a map of the pathophysiology of diabetes including, for example, the role of gluconeogenesis.

Have learners draw a map representing the pathophysiology of polyuria, polydipsia, and polyphagia.

Algorithm (10-15 min)

Ask groups of learners to develop a decision tree to identify actions needed when insulin reactions are suspected for a client on a twice-a-day regimen of NPH and regular insulin.

Ask groups of learners to develop a decision tree for both diabetic ketoacidosis and hyperglycemic hyperosmolar nonketotic syndrome. The tree should identify differences and similarities.

Journaling

Ask learners to develop a perioperative plan of care for the diabetic client. The plan of care should identify the differences between the diabetic and nondiabetic client going to surgery.

Ask learners to explain why diabetes mellitus results in pathophysiological changes in both the controlled and noncontrolled diabetic client.

Reflect on what the newly diagnosed IDDM client must feel, both physiologically and psychologically.

Campus lab/Clinical component (10-15 min)

Demonstrate some of the new aids for measuring blood glucose and insulin doses available for low-dose diabetic clients.

Have learners bring a variety of diabetic teaching tools and pamphlets to class or clinical to share with other learners.

Have learners pair up with a partner and teach the pathophysiology of diabetes in "lay" terms.

	Have learners prepare a 2-day meal plan using the exchange list and a 2-day plan using carbohydrate counting. **Structured controversy (15-20 min)** Diabetic clients should be candidates for pancreas or pancreas-kidney transplants. Third party payers should pay for these transplants. If more than one transplant is required, third party reimbursement should be discontinued. Diabetic clients should not be allowed to drive. **Numbered heads together (5-7 min)** Have even-numbered learners present information regarding a decision tree for the choice of oral hypoglycemics. Have odd-numbered learners present information regarding a decision tree for the choice of insulin preparation.	

TM 63-1

COMPARISON OF PITUITARY GLAND AND ADRENAL GLAND DISORDERS

	Pituitary Gland		**Adrenal Gland**	
	Excess	**Deficit**	**Excess**	**Deficit**
Common abnormal diagnostic laboratory test values				
Common abnormal radiologic tests				
Common clinical manifestations				
Therapeutic drug regimen				
Diet therapy				

CHAPTER 63

Case Study for the Client with Acromegaly and Hypophysectomy

A 56-year-old male client with acromegaly is scheduled to have a transphenoidal hypophysectomy. He has reported an increase in his hat, glove, and shoe size. He also discloses that he has had a problem with impotence. He is hypertensive and has hepatomegaly.

Questions

1. What information should you give this client before surgery?

2. During the postoperative period, what should you assess?

3. What are the possible complications of this surgery that you should be alert to?

4. What should you teach to this client before he goes home?

5. What expected outcomes are specific to this situation?

CHAPTER 64

Case Study for the Client with Graves' Disease

A 36-year-old female client returns to your nursing unit after having a subtotal thyroidectomy for Graves' disease. Her vital signs are stable, but she is complaining of circumoral tingling.

Questions

1. What laboratory data would you collect?

2. What additional physical assessment techniques would you perform?

3. What safety precautions would you institute?

4. What expected outcomes are specific to this situation?

CHAPTER 65

Case Study for the Client with Diabetes and Visual Impairment*

Your adult male client has had diabetes mellitus for several years. He takes 30 units of NPH with 10 units of regular insulin in the morning before breakfast and 20 units of NPH insulin before the evening meal. He has recently undergone laser therapy for treatment of diabetic retinopathy. He wants to be independent in insulin administration, and your assessment indicates that he has the intellectual ability to learn the needed skills.

Questions

1. List three methods for preventing both hypoglycemia and hyperglycemia that you would stress during your teaching sessions.

2. Discuss four ways of altering the environment to aid in the measurement of accurate insulin doses.

3. List five critical points that would be included in a teaching session on adaptive devices for use with insulin syringes.

*This Case Study is also available to students, along with web-based answer guidelines, in the *Critical Thinking Study Guide.*

UNIT 14 PROBLEMS OF PROTECTION: SKIN, HAIR, AND NAILS ■ Core Concepts Grid

Anatomy	Physiology	Pathophysiology	History	Physical Exam	Diagnostic Tests	Interventions	Pharmacology
• **Skin** Subcutaneous fat Epidermis Dermis • **Hair** • **Nails** • **Glands**	• **Protection** • **Regulation** Fluid balance Electrolyte balance Temperature • **Vitamin synthesis**	• **Inflammation** • **Infection** • **Tumors** • **Burns** Thermal Chemical Electrical	• **Client history** Dermatologic problems Medications Liver, gallbladder, renal disease • **Family history** Chronic skin prob-lems • **Social history** Occupation Nutritional status Sun exposure Age Race • **Risk for pressure ulcers**	• **Skin** Color Lesions Moisture Vascular markings Edema Intactness Tattoos Temperature Texture Turgor Depth (stage) of wound Drainage • **Hair/nails** Shape Distribution Texture	• **Cultures** • **Skin tests** Patch Scratch • **Biopsy**	• **Burn wound assessment** Depth Area Rule of Nines • **Burn fluid replacement formulas** • **Graft care** • **Care of burn wounds** • **Hypertrophy** • **Precautions for itching** • **Emotional support** • **Debridement** • **Wound dressings** • **Nutrition** • **Prevention of pressure ulcers** • **Skin/wound ongoing assessment**	• **Topical antibiotics** • **Topical antiin-flammatories** • **Keratolytic agents** • **Antipsoriasis agents** • **Debriding agents** • **Systemic antibiotics**

Unit 14 (Chapters 66-68)

Problems of Protection: Management of Clients with Problems of the Skin, Hair, and Nails

Learning Plan

Chapter 66: *Assessment of the Skin, Hair, and Nails*

Learning Outcomes	Learning Activities	Supplemental Resources
After reading this chapter, the student should be able to: 1. Compare the structure and function of the dermis with those of the epidermis. 2. Describe the integumentary changes associated with aging. 3. Use proper terminology to describe different skin lesions. 4. Describe techniques to assess skin changes in clients with dark skin. 5. Distinguish between normal variations and abnormal skin manifestations with regard to skin color, texture, warmth, and moisture. 6. Explain the role of melanocytes in determining skin color. 7. Describe the ABCD method of assessing skin lesions for cancer. 8. Prioritize educational needs for the client undergoing an excisional biopsy for a skin lesion.	**Think-pair-share (3-5 min)** Compare and contrast skin assessment of young and older clients. What treatment methods are available for aging skin? What is the purpose of sweat? Why is an assessment of the patient's medication history relative to an assessment of their skin? What is the difference in etiology between a primary skin lesion and a secondary lesion? What does hirsutism represent? What manifestations of pallor, erythema, and cyanosis will the nurse make on the dark-skinned client? **Campus lab/Clinical component** On a lab partner, demonstrate an assessment of the nails. Perform an assessment of the nails on your clinical client and report your findings.	**Internet resources** American Academy of Dermatology (Mature Skin) http://www.aad.org/pamphlets/agingskin.html

Chapter 67: *Interventions for Clients with Problems of the Skin and Nails*

Learning Outcomes	Learning Activities	Supplemental Resources
After reading this chapter, the student should be able to: 1. Prioritize nursing care for a client with dry skin. 2. Compare and contrast wound healing by first, second, and third intention.	**Think-pair-share exercises (3-5 min)** What are the typical patterns of skin eruptions seen with contact dermatitis and the rash seen with irritant contact dermatitis from exposure to chemicals? Describe the clinical characteristics of the varieties of malignant melanoma.	Worksheet 67-1 **Internet resources** The National Psoriasis Foundation http://www.psoriasis.org/

<table>
<tr>
<td>
3. Identify clients at risk for pressure ulcer development.
4. Plan an individualized strategy for pressure ulcer prevention for a specific client at increased risk.
5. Differentiate the clinical manifestations for stage I through stage IV pressure ulcers.
6. Prioritize the nursing interventions for a client with a stage III pressure ulcer.
7. Evaluate the effectiveness of interventions for pressure ulcer management.
8. Compare the clinical manifestations and modes of transmission for bacterial, viral, and fungal skin infections.
9. Explain the rationale for drug therapy for psoriasis.
10. Identify interventions for prevention of skin cancer.
11. Describe the clinical manifestations of melanoma.
12. Prioritize educational needs for the client undergoing an excisional biopsy for a skin lesion.
</td>
<td>
Identify some of the foods or drugs that cause common allergic reactions in the skin.
Compare and contrast the types of wounds to the types of wound healings (first intention in an incision, second intention in an abrasion, and third intention in an infected wound that has healed and can now be closed primarily).
Compare herpes simplex (type 1) with genital herpes (type 2) and with herpes zoster. Contrast the lesion's appearance, the symptoms, and the course of the illness (use Worksheet 37-1).
What data would support that an aesthetic plastic surgery was appropriate for a teenager?
What changes in a wound would signal possible wound infection or wound healing?
How can evaporative fluid losses with an open wound be estimated?
How can needed fluids be given to clients with open wounds?
What methods can be used to reduce body heat losses with an open wound?
What changes in self-concept are commonly seen with dermatological disease?
Why is dietary protein important in the healing of pressure ulcers and other wounds?
Describe the fluid and electrolyte disorders that may be seen in clients with skin problems, ranging from simple dryness to bullous skin disease.
Explain some positive and negative effects from the use of over-the-counter corticosteroid creams for various pruritic skin conditions.
Explain the use of skin oil supplementation in the treatment of psoriasis.
What are the effects of sun exposure and tanning booth exposure to the aging of skin and the development of skin cancer?
Describe the development of osteomyelitis from a pressure ulcer.
What are some surgical options for repair of pressure ulcers?
Describe the elimination diets for allergies.
What strategies are used for the client with pruritus?
Differentiate between pediculosis and scabies.
Explain the use of ultraviolet light therapy in the treatment of psoriasis.
</td>
<td>
The Wound Care Institute, Inc.
http://www.woundcare.org/

Wound, Ostomy and Continence Nurses Society
http://www.wocn.org/

Pressure Ulcers in Adults: Prediction and Prevention
Clinical practice guidelines online
http://www.ahcpr.gov/clinic/cpgonline.htm

Community resources
Have learners visit a local long-term care center and identify methods used to prevent pressure ulcers.
</td>
</tr>
</table>

Concept mapping (10-15 min)
Ask learners to map the pathophysiology of pressure ulcers. They should consider the risk of pressure, friction, and shearing forces.

Journaling
Ask learners to use their clients' various laboratory values to evaluate nutritional status and wound healing potential.
Identify some of the changes in lifestyle that occur with various skin problems such as eczema and psoriasis.
What role does malnutrition play in wound healing?

Campus lab/Clinical component
Ask learners to select a common hospital diet and evaluate if there are adequate dietary components to support wound healing.
Have groups of learners compare their clients' diets for adequate dietary support of wound healing.
Ask groups of learners to explore the costs of daily dressing changes versus use of skin protection aids such as hydrocolloidal dressings.
With a lab partner, construct a teaching plan for the client with genital herpes.

Structured controversy (10-15 min)
A client should be allowed to tell the insurance company that he or she has a problem requiring reconstructive surgery, which is covered by insurance, when it is really a cosmetic operation (e.g., rhinoplasty).
The use of fluorocarbons should be regulated because the incidence of skin cancer will continue to increase because the protective shielding of sunlight cannot occur without ozone.
The FDA should regulate the advertising of cosmetics.

Pairs check (5-10 min)
Demonstrate the correct technique to apply ointments. Consider the rationale for applying the ointment along the direction of the hair follicle and the impact the use of gloves has on the client.
Demonstrate nursing interventions to minimize development of pressure ulcers.

	Explore the costs of long-term dermatological diseases. **Algorithm (10-15 min)** Ask groups of learners to develop a decision tree for nursing interventions for an older client identified at risk for pressure ulcers. Refer learners to the Clinical Practice Guidelines Online.	

Chapter 68: *Interventions for Clients with Burns*

Learning Outcomes	Learning Activities	Supplemental Resources
After reading this chapter, the student should be able to: 1. Identify burn clients at risk for inhalation injury. 2. Compare and contrast the clinical manifestations of superficial, partial-thickness, and full-thickness burn injuries. 3. Explain the expected clinical manifestations of neural and hormonal compensation during the emergent phase of burn injury. 4. Calculate the total body surface area involved in a burn injury. 5. Prioritize nursing care for the client during the emergent phase of burn injury. 6. Use laboratory data and clinical manifestations to determine the effectiveness of fluid resuscitation during the emergent phase of burn injury. 7. Use the Parkland formula to establish the correct rate and timing of fluid replacement. 8. Prioritize nursing care for the client during the acute phase of burn injury. 9. Explain the alteration of nutritional needs for the burn client during the acute phase of burn injury. 10. Evaluate wound healing in the client during the acute phase of burn injury.	**Think-pair-share (3-5 min)** Identify the types of burn wound infections. Compare and contrast the topical agents used on burn wounds. Compare burn injury with other forms of trauma. Compare burn wound edema with edema from other causes, such as a sprained ankle, CHF, or cirrhosis. What changes are seen in a burn that indicate it is ready for skin grafting? What data indicate that a burn wound has become infected? Can a burn client and family learn a positive coping style while the client is hospitalized? What data would lead the nurse to suspect smoke inhalation? Discuss the phrase, "the client is the formula" when calculating IV fluid needs. How could a nurse work within this concept when infusing fluids and monitoring urine output during the emergent phase of the burn injury? What are the immune changes that occur with burn injury? Why are Jobst pressure garments used during burn wound healing? Why is smoke inhalation a greater risk in an enclosed building? Describe covering burn wounds with autologous microskin grafts.	**Internet resources** American Burn Association http://www.ameriburn.org/ Virtual Hospital – Burn Injuries http://www.vh.org/Patients/IHB/Surgery/BurnCenter/BurnInjury/burninjuriesTOC.html **Community resources** Have groups of learners participate in community endeavors to teach children fire safety. Have groups of learners identify fire safety mechanisms in their acute care facilities.

11. Compare and contrast pain management strategies for clients in the emergent and acute phases of burn injury. 12. Describe the characteristics of infected burn wounds. 13. Explain the positioning and range-of-motion interventions for the prevention of mobility problems in the client with burns. 14. Prioritize nursing care for the client during the rehabilitation phase of burn injury. 15. Discuss the potential psychosocial problems associated with burn injury.	Describe some strategies nurses might use to reduce the risk of burn injury in the community. **Numbered heads together (5-10 min)** Ask even-numbered learners to identify some pharmacological pain management strategies for the burn client whose wounds are being debrided. Ask odd-numbered learners to identify some nonpharmacologic pain management strategies for the burn client whose wounds are being debrided. **Journaling** Discuss the risks and advantages of early excision of eschar (within 48 hours after burn) and grafting. Consider bleeding potential, anesthetic risk, hemodynamic instability, shortened healing time, and decreased incidence of complications related to open wounds and immobility. Explain why pain medications are given intravenously to burn victims in the initial stages of burn recovery. Explain why antibiotics are seldom given to a burn client until there are signs of a wound infection. Identify methods of teaching a burn client how to resume a normal diet once the wounds have closed and nutritional needs are less. **Concept mapping (10-15 min)** Ask learners to map the pathophysiology of electrical burns. It should include how the electricity must exit the body through a "ground' and that it burns everything along its path. **Group learning (5-10 min)** Ask groups of learners to identify some of the changes in lifestyle that occur following burn injury, such as immediate changes in family roles and long-term changes in work. Have learners pass their responses to a second group who should add any additional items. Ask groups of learners to calculate the calories needed by a 70-kg man after a 40% burn injury. Discuss methods to provide these calories, such as adding supplements to the regular foods, extra feedings, hyperalimentation, and tube feeding.	

	Ask groups of learners to calculate the fluid needs for a 79-kg man with a 50% TBSA burn. How much fluid is needed in the first 8 hours after injury? How much after 16 hours? Consider the time of injury in the calculation of the fluid needed for the first 8 hours. **Campus lab/Clinical component** Manage care for clients who are being treated with flotation beds. **Structured controversy (10-15 min)** A severely burned client should be allowed to die rather than go through painful recovery. Laws should be passed to protect innocent victims of burns (e.g., it should be illegal to smoke in bed, to store gas in nonmetal containers, and to have matches near children).	

TM 67-1

COMPARISON OF HERPES

	Herpes Simplex (1)	**Herpes Simplex (2)**	**Herpes Zoster**
Appearance of lesion			
Clinical manifestations			
Course of illness			
Drug therapy			

CHAPTER 67

Case Study for the Client with a Candida *Skin Infection*

You are assigned to make a home visit and perform an initial nursing assessment on a 92-year-old woman with a diagnosis of right lower lobe pneumonia. The client is bedridden and confused, requiring the constant care of her 68-year-old daughter, who lives with the client. While completing a head-to-toe skin assessment, the daughter explains that her mother "can't control her urine." On removing the adult briefs, you note that the client grimaces. The perineal area is inflamed with denuded areas of skin that are open and weeping. A red papular rash is also observed in the gluteal fold and groin areas.

Questions

1. What assessment information do you need to document?

2. What additional skin assessment data do you need to collect and document?

3. What priority nursing actions do you need to implement?

4. What expected outcomes would be specific to this situation?

CHAPTER 68

Case Study for the Client with a Burn Injury

A 45-year-old male client is admitted to the burn unit after rescue from a house fire. He is incoherent and has burns of the face, head, neck, circumferential bilateral arms and legs, and one half of the anterior chest. Carbon particles are present around the nose and mouth. He is short of breath and complains of pain in the face and arms.

Questions

1. What initial physical assessment techniques and interventions should be done during the primary survey?

2. Once the patient is stabilized, what ongoing assessment parameters should be undertaken during the emergent phase of injury?

3. Discuss actual and potential problems with interventions that may be done during the acute phase of burn injury.

4. During the rehabilitation phase of burn injury, what teaching parameters should be implemented for the patient and his family?

PROBLEMS OF EXCRETION: RENAL/URINARY ■ Core Concepts Grid

Anatomy	Physiology	Pathophysiology	History	Physical Exam	Diagnostic Tests	Interventions	Pharmacology
• **Macro-structures** Kidneys Ureters Bladder Urethra • **Micro-structures** Cortex Medulla Pelvis Glomerulus Nephron	• **Regulation** Water balance Waste products Acid-base balance • **Synthesis of hormones** Erythropoietin Renin Activated vitamin D • **Glomerular filtration**	• **Obstruction** • **Inflammation** • **Infection** • **Trauma** • **Tumors** • **Metabolic acidosis**	• **Client history** Past renal problems Difficulty with urination Change in urinary elimination pattern Pain Hypertension • **Family history** Diabetes mellitus Hypertension • **Social history** Alcohol/drug use Occupation Age	• **Skin** Color/turgor Moisture • **Eyes** Conjunctiva • **Mouth** Moisture/color Ulceration • **Chest** Shape Pulsation • **Periphery** Color Hair distribution Striae/edema Pulses/rashes • **Abdomen** Striae/tenderness over kidney Bruits over renal artery	• **Urinalysis** • **Specific gravity** • **Sediment** • **Serum creatinine** • **Blood urea nitrogen (BUN)** • **Uric acid** • **Scans** • **Renal arteriogram** • **Kidney, ureter, and bladder (KUB)** • **Sonograms** • **Intravenous pyelography (IVP)** • **Biopsy** • **Creatinine clearance** • **Serum pH** • **Cystoscopy**	• **Fluid regulation** • **Dialysis** Hemodialysis Peritoneal dialysis Continuous ambulatory peritoneal dialysis (CAPD) • **Renal transplantation** • **Extracorporeal shock wave lithotripsy (ESWL)** • **AV fistula** • **AV shunt** • **Therapeutic diet** • **Fluids, as appropriate** • **Lithotripsy** • **Health teaching** • **Bladder training** • **Skin care** • **Urinary catherter care**	• **Diuretics** • **Anti-inflammatories** • **Antibiotics** • **Immunosuppressive agents** • **Calcium replacement agents** • **Hormone replacement agents** • **Chelating agents** • **Phosphorus-binding agents** • **Anticholinergics** • **Skin barrier topical agents**

Unit 15 (Chapters 69-72)

Problems of Excretion: Management of Clients with Problems of the Renal/Urinary System

Learning Plan

Chapter 69: *Assessment of the Renal/Urinary System*

Learning Outcomes	Learning Activities	
After reading this chapter, the student should be able to: 1. Compare and contrast kidney function with functions of the ureters, bladder, and urethra. 2. Describe the roles of the afferent and efferent arterioles in glomerular filtration. 3. Explain the influence of antidiuretic hormone and aldosterone on urine formation and composition. 4. Describe age-related changes in the renal/urinary system. 5. Use laboratory data to distinguish between dehydration and renal impairment. 6. Describe how to obtain a sterile urine specimen from a client with a Foley catheter. 7. Identify teaching priorities for a client who needs to obtain a 24-hour specimen. 8. Identify teaching priorities for a client who needs to obtain a "clean catch" urine specimen. 9. Describe the correct techniques to use in physically assessing the renal system. 10. Prioritize nursing care for the client during the first 24 hours following a renal arteriogram.	**Think-pair-share (3-5 min)** Identify glomerular filtration, tubular reabsorption, and tubular secretion and their roles in removing electrolytes, fluid, acids, and metabolic waste products from the kidney. Identify renal/urinary laboratory changes (in BUN, CBC, uric acid, creatinine, and electrolytes) that occur in older adults. How is red blood cell formation related to a study of the kidney? How does aging affect the renal/urinary system? Why should urine specimens be delivered to the lab as soon as possible? Why is a "clean catch" urine specimen preferred? What abnormal outcomes can be discovered from an intravenous pyelography? What does the term *retrograde* mean in relation to urine flow, and what would be the purpose of a retrograde exam? What is the relationship between blood pressure and the renal system? What does the color of urine indicate? What are the nursing responsibilities in caring for clients undergoing diagnostic testing of the urinary system? **Campus lab/Clinical component** With a partner, explain the procedures for obtaining a clean catch urine. Have learners identify the many things that could go wrong during a 24-hour urine collection and plan interventions to keep these from happening. The "client" asks, "Why if it's my kidneys, does my back hurt?" Teach a partner about the anatomy of the renal system.	

	Practice catheterization of clients. Practice collecting urine specimens from Foley catheter systems, urinals, and bedpans. Vary the specimens for them to practice testing for sugar, ketones, and other components (for instance, add D_5W to various colored-water specimens). **Pairs check (5-10 min)** Give several samples of various intake and output amounts and have students calculate totals for an 8- and a 24-hour period.	

Chapter 70: *Interventions for Clients with Urinary Problems*

Learning Outcomes	Learning Activities	Supplemental Resource
After reading this chapter, the student should be able to: 1. Describe the clinical manifestations of cystitis. 2. Prioritize educational needs for a person at risk for cystitis. 3. Compare and contrast the pathophysiology and manifestations of stress incontinence, urge incontinence, overflow incontinence, mixed incontinence, and functional incontinence. 4. Prioritize educational needs for the client taking sulfonamide antibiotics for a urinary tract infection. 5. Describe the techniques to assess pelvic floor strength in the client who is experiencing some incontinence. 6. Explain the proper application of exercises to strengthen pelvic floor muscles. 7. Explain the drug therapy for different types of incontinence. 8. Prioritize nursing care for the client with renal colic.	**Think-pair-share (3-5 min)** What is the role of calcium intake in the client with kidney stones? What is the most common pathogen in infectious cystitis? What is the relationship between vaginal contraceptives and cystitis? What is the role of estrogen in treating estrogen-depletion urethritis? Compare the urinary incontinence and urinary retention that occur in older clients and younger clients. What happens to bladder function following removal of an indwelling catheter? Should people who are incontinent be catheterized? Does it aid in preventing the development of pressure ulcers? What are the risks? Identify teaching strategies for preventing UTIs in clients. What questions would help determine if a client has a problem with incontinence? What is the association between social isolation and urinary incontinence? How do cranberry juice and blueberry juice prevent urinary tract infections?	**Internet resource** National Kidney and Urologic Disease Information Clearinghouse – Urinary Tract Infection in Adults http://www.niddk.nih.gov/health/urolog/pubs/utiadult/utiadult.htm

9. Describe the common clinical manifestations of bladder cancer. 10. Develop a teaching plan for a client who has had a urinary diversion for bladder cancer.	Why is vitamin C administered for decreasing urinary pH? In clients with renal calculi, what does oliguria progressing to anuria suggest? How does lithotripsy work in the treatment of renal calculi? **Concept mapping (10-15 min)** Describe the development of urine incontinence devices for women. Describe the development of renal calculi. **Pairs check (5-7 min)** Ask learners to role play assessment of the renal and urinary systems with a provided health history. **Algorithm (10-15 min)** Ask learners to develop a decision tree for treating incontinence. **Numbered heads together (5-10 min)** Ask even-numbered learners to develop quality assurance improvement standards related to indwelling catheter care. Ask odd-numbered learners to identify the knowledge and skills unlicensed assistive personnel must have when caring for a client with an indwelling catheter. **Group learning (10-20 min)** Ask groups of learners to identify clients at risk of developing urinary tract infections and possible interventions to minimize the risk. Ask groups of learners to design a perioperative care plan for the client undergoing surgical treatment for stress urinary incontinence. Ask groups of learners to design a care plan for clients with urinary retention, urinary incontinence, and chronic urinary tract infections. Ask learners to develop a care plan for the client using vaginal cone therapy. **Journaling** Ask learners to identify the various treatment for bladder cancer and the various types of continent urinary diversion options, and describe the use of artificial urinary sphincter for treatment of male incontinence following postprostatectomy incontinence.	

Chapter 71: *Interventions for Clients with Renal Disorders*

Learning Outcomes	Learning Activities	Supplemental Resources
After reading this chapter, the student should be able to: 1. Prioritize nursing care needs for the client with polycystic kidney disease. 2. Describe the clinical manifestations of hydronephrosis. 3. Identify clients at risk for pyelonephritis. 4. Use laboratory data and clinical manifestations to determine the effectiveness of therapy for pyelonephritis. 5. Compare and contrast the pathophysiology and clinical manifestations of acute glomerulonephritis and nephritic syndrome. 6. Prioritize nursing care needs for the client during the first 24 hours after nephrectomy. 7. Explain how diabetic nephropathy can affect glucose metabolism and control in the client with diabetes mellitus. 8. Develop a teaching plan for the client who has had a nephrectomy for renal cell carcinoma.	**Think-pair-share (3-5 min)** What questions should be asked when obtaining a sexual history from a client with renal urinary disease? Identify the type and site of action of diuretics in the renal tubules (use Worksheets 71-1 and 71-2). What is the relationship between hypertension and polycystic disease? Why is hematuria a symptom of polycystic disease? What are the symptoms of pyelonephritis? Why is pyelonephritis more likely to occur following placement of a urinary catheter? What symptoms would suggest that pyelonephritis is progressing to renal failure? What is the relationship between pulmonary tuberculosis and renal tuberculosis? What are the differences in clinical manifestations of glomerulonephritis in the older adult population? Why does hypertension accompany glomerulonephritis? Differentiate acute glomerulonephritis from chronic glomerulonephritis. Why would the nurse expect to see proteinuria in the urinalysis of the client with glomerulonephritis? Why would electrolyte levels be abnormal in the client with decreased renal function? Why does diabetes mellitus lead to end stage renal disease? How is the diagnosis of renal trauma made? **Journaling** Describe the psychosocial impact of polycystic kidney disease as an inherited disorder. **Group learning** Have groups of learners develop a 2-day diet plan for the client with nephrosis. Include information for the client about necessary modifications such as sodium restriction.	Worksheet 71-1 Worksheet 71-2 **Internet resources** Virtual Hospital Pathology of Kidney: Glomerulonephritis http://www.vh.org/Providers/Textbooks/GN/GNHP.htm National Kidney and Urologic Disease Information Clearinghouse http://www.niddk.nih.gov/health/urolog/urolog.htm

	Concept mapping Contrast hydronephrosis, hydroureter, and urethral stricture by mapping the pathophysiological changes these disorders produce. Draw a map of the development of pyelonephritis. Have learners include in their map the progression from acute to chronic pyelonephritis. **Campus lab/Clinical component** Identify the electrolyte results the nurse would expect to find in the client with glomerulonephritis. What would the nurse expect to see in the urinalysis of the client with pyelonephritis? Develop a dietary plan for protein replacement in the client with nephritic syndrome.	

Chapter 72: *Interventions for Clients with Chronic and Acute Renal Failure*

Learning Outcomes	Learning Activities	Supplemental Resources
After reading this chapter, the student should be able to: 1. Compare and contrast the pathophysiology and causes of chronic renal failure and acute renal failure. 2. Identify clients at risk for development of acute renal failure. 3. Identify clients at risk for development of chronic renal failure. 4. Use laboratory data and clinical assessment to determine the effectiveness of therapy for renal failure. 5. Discuss interventions to prevent acute renal failure. 6. Prioritize the nursing care needs of the client in acute renal failure. 7. Compare the clinical manifestations of stage I, stage II, and stage III chronic renal failure.	**Think-pair-share (3-5 min)** Identify stages the client and family must go through while adapting to the diagnosis of chronic renal failure. Identify the types of antacids to be used for various electrolyte imbalances seen in renal failure. Describe the processes of continuous arteriovenous hemofiltration (CAVH) and continuous arteriovenous hemodialysis (CAVHD). How do the diet restrictions for ESRD affect diet intake and bowel elimination (constipation)? Compare the advantages and disadvantages of the types of dialyses as they affect the client's quality of life. Discuss the rationale for early renal transplantation for the client with diabetic nephropathy. Identify the effects of ESRD and dialysis on the stunted growth of children and the effect that they may have on the client when he or she reaches adulthood. Identify the predicted and actual quality-of-life changes that occur following renal transplantation.	**Internet resources** End Stage Renal Disease http://www.niddk.nih.gov/health/kidney/pubs/esrd/esrd.htm Hypertension, Dialysis & Clinical Nephrology http://www.hdcn.com/ National Kidney Foundation http://www.kidney.org/ The Kidney Transplant Dialysis Association http://www.ultranet.com/~ktda/ The Nephron Information Center http://www.nephron.com/kidneydisease.html United States Renal Data System http://www.usrds.org/

8. Discuss the mechanisms of peritoneal dialysis and hemodialysis as renal replacement therapies. 9. Prioritize the nursing care needs of the client with ESRD. 10. Prioritize teaching needs for the client using CAPD. 11. Prioritize teaching needs for the clients with a permanent vascular access for long-term hemodialysis. 12. Compare and contrast the dietary modifications needed for the client undergoing hemodialysis with those for the client undergoing peritoneal dialysis. 13. Plan prevention strategies for the complications of peritoneal dialysis. 14. Discuss the criteria for kidney donation. 15. Prioritize nursing care needs for the client during the first 24 hours after kidney transplantation.	What pathophysiological changes lead to fatigue and activity intolerance in the client with ESRD? How does uremic frost develop? Identify some body image changes associated with dialysis and transplantation (e.g., clients undergoing dialysis often draw the dialysis machine as a part of their body) and nursing interventions to help clients accommodate to the changes. Identify ways to encourage food intake despite the metallic taste characteristic of renal failure. What are the effects of diet restrictions for ESRD on the adult in relation to muscle strength and energy? Explain why potassium salt substitutes should be avoided by clients with ESRD. Identify the types of foods to be avoided and those to be encouraged for the client on a low-sodium, low-protein, or low-potassium diet. How can nurses make these boring diets more interesting? What are the dosing differences of medications given to clients with ESRD? Describe the administration time of medications for clients being dialyzed. Describe the administration of cyclosporine for kidney transplantation clients and any precautions the nurse must take with liquid cyclosporine. Describe the principles use in the various types of dialysis. Why are clients at increased risk of HIV and hepatitis infection during hemodialysis? **Group learning (5-10 min)** Ask groups of learners to identify causes of acute renal failure and nursing interventions to prevent ART from happening to clients while under their care. **Concept mapping (10-15 min)** Identify how end-stage renal disease affects the client and family members. Map the long-term complications of renal transplantation.	**Community resources** Have groups of learners spend a day in a dialysis unit. Invite a person undergoing dialysis to come and speak to the class.

Numbered head together (5-7 min)

Ask even-numbered learners to describe the use of Epoetin alfa (recombinant human erythropoietin) for treatment of ESRD anemia. Ask odd-numbered learners to describe the side effects of NSAIDs in the development of acute renal failure.

Structured controversy (5-10 min)

People with inherited disorders that progress to ESRD should not be allowed to bear children.

The government should be responsible to provide the dollars needed to treat ESRD.

Terminally ill clients who develop renal failure should not be dialyzed.

Potential organ donors should be paid money for organ donation.

ESRD clients who overeat, over-drink, or fail to take care of the cannula are really committing suicide.

A potential donor who does not want to donate an organ should be forced to donate anyway to save a life.

Journaling

Assign learners to investigate the costs of hemodialysis in a health care setting or in the home, and of peritoneal dialysis in a health care setting or via CAPD, and of kidney transplantation.

Identify some effects of diet restrictions on the coping abilities of clients with ESRD. Consider clients who cannot eat at fast food restaurants or cannot go out and indulge themselves in food or drink without ill effects.

Can the renal transplant client return to work?

Identify some ethical issues to be decided when discontinuing dialysis therapy.

Campus lab/Clinical component

Prepare and administer a Kayexalate enema.

Visit a dialysis center for a day.

TM 71-1

NEPHRON UNIT

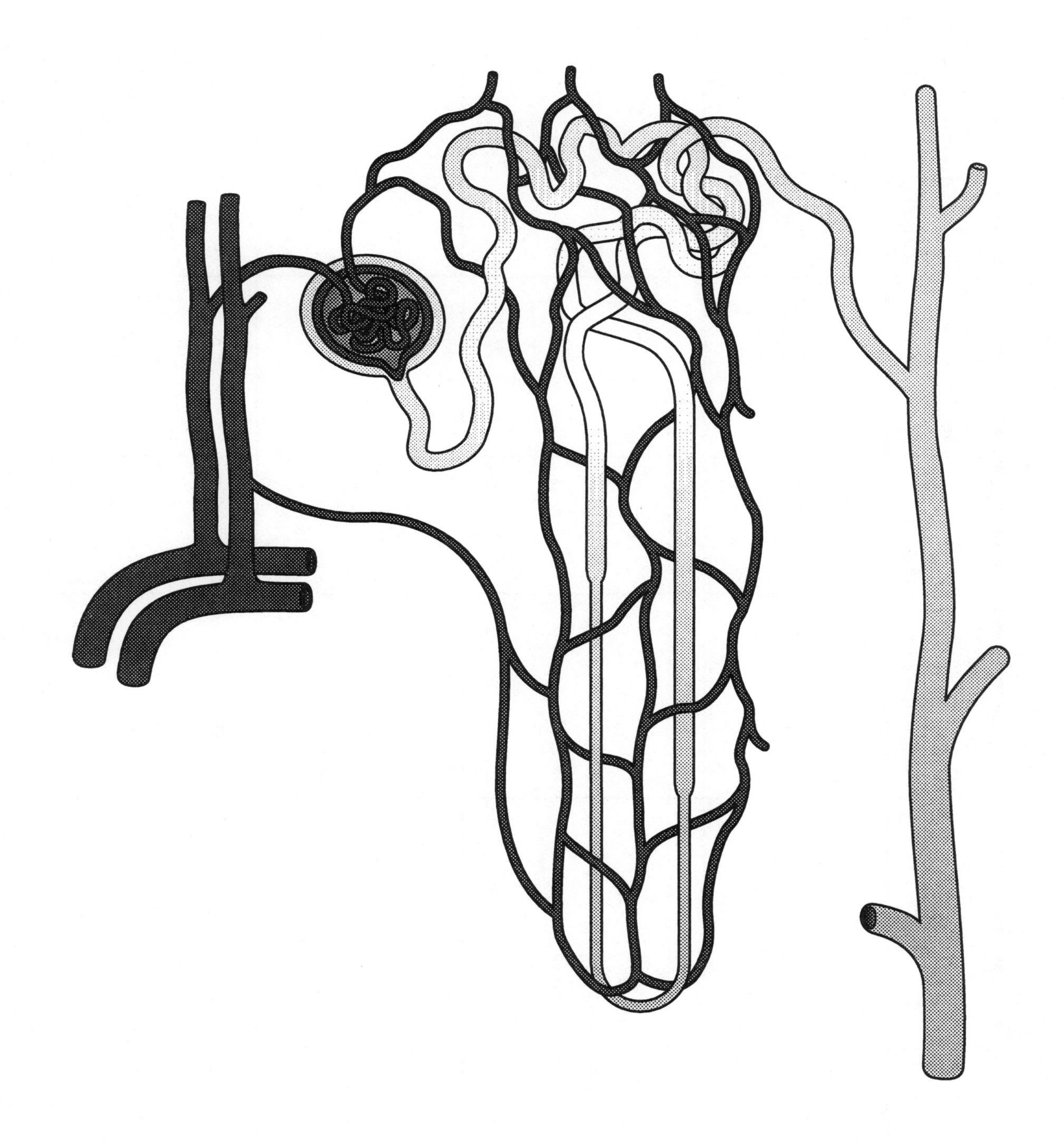

TM 71-2

DIURETICS

	Drug/ Classification	Action	Indications for Use	Side/Adverse Effects	Nursing Indications
Carbonic Anhydrase Inhibitors Acetazolamide (Diamox)					
Thiazides Chlorothiazide (Diuril) Methyclothiazide (Enduron)					
Loop Furosemide (Lasix) Ethacrynic acid (Edecrin) Bumetanide (Bumex)					
Potassium Sparing Amiloride (Midamor) Spironolactone (Aldactone) Triamterene (Dyrenium)					

CHAPTER 70

Case Study for the Client with Urinary Incontinence

A 88-year-old woman is in the hospital for pneumonia. She is responding well to antibiotic therapy, but you notice she only makes small amounts of concentrated urine; often she is incontinent. When you try to encourage her to drink (as prescribed), she says, "Oh honey, I can't drink that. If I do I won't be able to get to the bathroom in time."

Questions

1. What is the client probably thinking that led her to the response she gave you?

2. How important is it for the client to force fluids? Why?

3. Other than explaining why she needs an increased fluid intake, what other interventions could you discuss with the client?

CHAPTER 71

Case Study for the Client with Diabetic Nephropathy

A client has had diabetes for 15 years and has recently been diagnosed with diabetic nephropathy. She tells you, "Well, now I got the disease in my kidneys. There isn't anything I can do now . . . I may as well give up. Dialysis, here I come, ready or not!"

Questions

1. How would you initially respond to her?

2. What would you say to her about dialysis?

3. What resources could you refer her to?

CHAPTER 72

Case Study for the Client with Acute Renal Failure

A 77-year-old female nursing home resident is admitted to the medical-surgical unit with a temperature of 100.8° F, a pulse rate of 96, respirations of 22, and a blood pressure of 176/94. The nursing home staff reports that she has been lethargic and has had a decline in urine output for the past 2 days. Her medical history includes hypertension and arthritis. Her current medications consist of ibuprofen 400 mg PO TID and captopril 25 mg PO BID. You are about to begin your initial assessment of this client.

Questions

1. What risk factors possibly predispose this client to acute renal failure?

2. What measures could be taken to avoid ARF in this client?

3. What circumstances would cause the BUN/creatinine ratio to be elevated in this client?

UNIT 16 PROBLEMS OF REPRODUCTION ■ Core Concepts Grid

Anatomy	Physiology	Pathophysiology	History	Physical Exam	Diagnostic Tests	Interventions	Pharmacology
• **Female** Ovaries Fallopian tubes Uterus Vagina • **Male** Penis Scrotum Testes Ducts • **Breasts**	• **Procreation** • **Nurturing** • **Sexual pleasure** • **Urinary elimination**	• **Infection** • **Obstruction** • **Inflammation** • **Tumors**	• **Client history** Past problems Contraceptives Obstetric history Self-examination Breast Testes Difficult/painful urination Menstrual history Erectile dysfunction Renal/endocrine dysfunction Hypertension • **Family history** Cancer Thyroid Diabetes • **Social history** Sexual history Alcohol use Smoking Exposure to sexually transmitted disease (STDs) Age Race	• **Skin/hair distribution** • **Skin ulceration/ rashes/color** • **Discharge** Vagina Penis Nipple • **Hernia** • **Breastss** Size Shape Masses	• **Mammography** • **Ultrasonography** • **Pap smear** • **Estrogen levels** • **Androgen levels** • **Venereal Disease Research Labora-tory (VDRL) test** • **Fluorescent Tre-ponemal Antibody Absorption (FTA-ABS) test** • **Gram stain** • **Acid phosphate** • **Prostate-specific antigen (PSA)** • **Carcinoembryonic antigen (CEA)**	• **Radiation ther-apy** • **Client education** Self-examination Breast Testes Safer sex Hormone replace-ment therapy (HRT) Kegel exercises • **Bladder irriga-tions** • **Urinary catheter care** Foley (3-way) Suprapubic • **Penile implants** • **Postoperative care and moni-toring for com-plications (e.g., hemorrhage)** • **Sperm banking** • **Emotional sup-port** • **Health teaching**	• **Antibiotics** • **Antivirals** • **Antiprotozoals** • **Antifungals** • **Hormone replacement therapy** • **Anti-impotence agents** • **Chemothera-peutic agents**

Unit 16 (Chapters 73-77)

Problems of Reproduction: Management of Clients with Problems of the Reproductive System

Learning Plan

Chapter 73: *Assessment of the Reproductive System*

Learning Outcomes	Learning Activities	Supplemental Resources
After studying this chapter, the student should be able to: 1. Review the anatomy and physiology of the reproductive system. 2. Discuss the components of a health history for reproductive health problems using Gordon's Functional Health Patterns. 3. Interpret common reproductive diagnostic tests. 4. Describe the client preparation for common reproductive diagnostic tests. 5. Develop a teaching plan for clients undergoing endoscopic studies for reproductive health problems. 6. Explain the importance of selected reproductive tests in promoting and maintaining health (e.g., mammogram).	**Think-pair-share (3-5 min)** What information should be collected related to sexual functioning while collecting a health history—particularly a reproductive health history? What impact does smoking have on sexual performance? What effect might obesity have on sexual functioning? Identify foods that may contribute to the development of problems in the genitoreproductive system, such as caffeine and fibrocystic breast changes or a high-fat diet and breast or uterine cancer. Identify drugs that may cause sexual dysfunction and their alternatives. Compare and contrast physical changes during the aging process related to sexuality. What nursing interventions are indicated for the client who is going to take a fertility drug to stimulate ovulation but is worried about the risk of multiple births? Identify alternate positions for sexual intercourse for clients with back pain, ostomies, heart and respiratory diseases, and paralysis. What is the rationale for protection of the genitals during x-rays? What are some methods for encouraging clients to routinely have a Pap smear? Describe various methods of birth control: condoms, vasectomy, tubal ligation, hysterectomy, cervical cap, IUD, birth control pills, etc. Describe methods for protecting the male and female genitalia during sports activities.	**Internet resources** Association of Women's Health, Obstetric, and Neonatal Nurses http://www.awhonn.org/ Oncology Nursing Society http://www.ons.org/ Association of Reproductive Health Professionals http://www.arhp.org/arhpframe.html Reproductive Health Online http://www.reproline.jhu.edu/ CDC's Reproductive Health: Information Source http://www.cdc.gov/nccdphp/drh/wh_women.htm **Community resources** Invite an oncology clinical specialist to discuss current treatments for cancer of the genitoreproductive system in men and women. Visit a local health department's clinic for Reproductive Health. Determine types of problems that are treated (e.g., birth control) and those services that are referred to another care provider (a client with cervical cancer following an abnormal screening). Have learners informally poll clients in a public place (e.g., shopping mall) about their self-screening practices (BSE, TSE).

Pairs check (10-15 min)

Role-play conducting a history and physical examination for gynecological client.

Role-play teaching teenagers about condoms.

Role-play teaching various forms of birth control to males and females.

Concept mapping (10-15 min)

Map the anatomy and physiology of the male and female reproductive systems.

Map the effect of the endocrine system on genitoreproductive tissue (e.g., FSH, LH).

Map the relationship among human sexuality, body image, and self-esteem.

Make a decision tree for determining whether an elderly couple should room together in a nursing home.

Map the male and female reproductive processes and insert contraceptive methods at the point(s) where they prevent conception.

Journaling (10-15 min)

Have learners compare and contrast the portrayal of female and male bodies in painting and sculpture throughout the centuries.

Ask a group of learners to investigate various cultures, with emphasis on their beliefs, attitudes, and practices of feminine hygiene.

How can cancer support groups be used for clients with reproductive organ cancers?

Structured controversy (10-15 min)

Should abortion be legal for all women? Should tax dollars be used to pay for them?

Should there be laws mandating sterilization? Consider mentally retarded people and women with several out-of-wedlock pregnancies who are on welfare.

Should genital self-examination (BSE, TSE, and VSE) be included in public school curricula?

Victims of sexual abuse should receive compensation from their abuser.

Chapter 74: *Interventions for Clients with Breast Disorders*

Learning Outcomes	Learning Activities	Supplemental Resources
After studying this chapter, the student should be able to: 1. Describe the three-pronged approach to early detection of breast masses: mammography, clinical breast examination, and breast self-examination (BSE). 2. Teach a client how to do BSE. 3. Explain the options available to a woman at high genetic risk for breast cancer. 4. Compare and contrast assessment findings associated with benign and malignant breast lesions. 5. Analyze assessment data to determine priority nursing diagnoses and collaborative problems for a woman with breast cancer. 6. Develop a plan of care for a client with breast cancer. 7. Discuss the psychosocial aspects related to having breast cancer and undergoing surgery for breast cancer. 8. Formulate a community-based teaching plan for clients undergoing surgery for breast cancer.	**Think-pair-share (3-5 min)** Have learners complete TM 74-1 prior to class; compare answers. **Numbered heads together (7-10 min)** After comparing TM 74-1 answers, ask half of the group to compare and contrast advantages and disadvantages of different types of mastectomies. Ask the remaining group to compare and contrast nursing considerations for the different types of mastectomies. **Think-pair-share (3-5 min)** What interventions can be used to help women who do not practice breast self-examination to begin routinely doing so? Identify why some women but not others may desire breast reconstruction. What are some interventions for clients to minimize development of lymph edema following breast cancer surgery? What are some reasons that women choose breast augmentation to increase breast size? What are the common complaints of clients who have received silicone breast implants? How does the nutritional status of a client affect the success of chemotherapy? Identify some issues created by conflicting results about the effects of birth control pills on the development of breast cancer. Explain why tamoxifen (Nolvadex) is effective in the treatment of breast cancer. How can hair loss from chemotherapy be prevented? Explain why chemotherapy is beneficial after breast cancer surgery for which metastasis has not been found. Identify the reasons why many women may have phantom breast experiences following mastectomy. **Pairs check (10-15 min)** Practice postmastectomy exercises.	**Transparency master** TM 74-1 Comparison of surgical procedures for breast cancer **Internet resources** Y-ME http://www.y-me.org/ Info: Breast Cancer http://www.infobreastcancer.cyberus.ca/ HealthTalk Interactive: Breast Cancer Education Network http://www.healthtalk.com/bcen/ CancerNet: Screening for Breast Cancer http://cancernet.nci.nih.gov/cgi-bin/srchcgi.exe?DBID=pdq&TYPE=search&UID=280+01955&ZFILE=patient&SFMT=pdq_scrprv/1/0/0 National Breast Cancer Foundation, Inc. http://www.nationalbreastcancer.org/index32.htm **Community resources** Assign learners to assess the availability of health information and diagnostic screening facilities related to cancer of the female reproductive system in their immediate area. Invite a client who has had a mastectomy, ostomy, or amputation to discuss body image changes and coping mechanisms. Invite a member of Reach to Recovery to discuss the physical, psychosocial, and rehabilitative needs of the client who has undergone a mastectomy. Y-ME National Organization for Breast Cancer Information and Support: 800-221-2141. Breast cancer survivors provide information, counseling, and referrals to treatment centers and support and self-help groups.

	Concept mapping (10-15 min) Make an algorithm evaluating a woman's need for breast reconstruction following mastectomy. For instance, is the woman content to be rid of the cancer or is there a need to have the breast tissue reconstructed to retain femininity? **Structured controversy (10-15 min)** Should women who have ruptured silicone breast implants be compensated for the cost, pain, and chronic health problems resulting from disseminated silicone?	Have learners visit a local high school and present concepts about BSE to girls in the upper class levels. Enlist the help of the local health department.

Chapter 75: *Interventions for Clients with Gynecologic Problems*

Learning Outcomes	Learning Activities	Supplemental Resources
After studying this chapter, the student should be able to: 1. Compare and contrast common menstrual cycle disorders. 2. Discuss common assessment findings associated with menopause. 3. Develop a teaching plan for a client with a vaginal inflammation or infection. 4. Prioritize postoperative care for the client undergoing an anterior and/or posterior repair. 5. Analyze assessment data for clients with leiomyomas to determine nursing diagnoses and collaborative problems. 6. Formulate a plan of care for a client undergoing a hysterectomy. 7. Identify the risk factors for gynecologic cancers. 8. Discuss the psychosocial issues associated with gynecologic cancers. 9. Explain the purpose of radiation and chemotherapy for clients with gynecologic cancers. 10. Develop a community-based plan of care for clients with gynecologic cancers.	**Think-pair-share (3-5 min)** What role or influence does rigorous exercise have on the menstrual cycle? Describe the relationship of the introduction of super absorbent, long-term tampons and the increased number of toxic shock syndrome cases. Compare the various conditions that arise from the relaxation of pelvic muscles. Compare the advantages and disadvantages of douching. Discuss methods to effectively assess substance abuse in a hospitalized client. List several ways to effectively communicate with a client who is suspected of abusing a substance. How does the nutritional status of a client affect the success of chemotherapy? What diet changes may aid vaginitis prophylaxis? How is goserelin acetate (Zoladex) used for treatment of endometriosis? How can hair loss from chemotherapy be prevented?	**Internet resources** OB/GYN Net: Menopause & Perimenopause http://www.obgyn.net/meno/meno.asp Menopause Online http://www.menopause-online.com/ Menopause and Beyond http://www.oxford.net/~tishy/beyond.html Women & Menopause http://www.womenandmenopause.com/ Hyster Sisters: Hysterectomy Support http://www.hystersisters.com/ All About Pap Tests http://www.gyncancer.com/pap-test.html Eyes on the Prize: Living with GYN Cancer http://www.eyesontheprize.org/links/news.html

	Pairs check (10-15 min) Prepare and administer a sitz bath. Administer perineal care. Give an enema. Demonstrate and discuss various types of vaginal specula. Role-play describing how to insert a pessary. (Have sample pessaries available.) Practice vulvar and vaginal irrigations on a model. **Numbered heads together (7-10 min)** Ask half the group to describe the use of paclitaxel (Taxol) as a chemotherapeutic agent for treatment of ovarian cancer. The other half should describe the use of the drug ifosfamide (Ifex) for male clients with testicular cancer. (See Chapter 76.) **Concept mapping (10-15 min)** Map the concepts of two types of substance abuse. **Journaling (10-15 min)** Have learners investigate female sexual mutilation practices (for celibacy until marriage). **Structured controversy (10-15 min)** Too many hysterectomies are carried out unnecessarily.	**Community resources** Invite an OB/GYN health care provider (MD or Nurse Practitioner) to visit the class to discuss frequently treated gynecologic problems. Emphasize the nurse's role. Invite a client who has experienced a "surgical" menopause (hysterectomy and/or oophorectomy) to discuss adjustments and treatment.

Chapter 76: *Interventions for Male Clients with Reproductive Problems*

Learning Outcomes	Learning Activities	Supplemental Resources
After studying this chapter, the student should be able to: 1. Describe common physical assessment findings for the client with benign prostatic hyperplasia (BPH). 2. Discuss options for nonsurgical and surgical management of the client with BPH. 3. Develop a postoperative plan of care for a client undergoing a transurethral resection of the prostate (TURP).	**Think-pair-share (3-5 min)** Complete TM 76-1 prior to class; compare answers. Determine lab tests and values that differentiate between BPH and prostatic cancer. Which tests would differentiate between physical and psychological causes of impotence? What interventions can be used to help men who do not practice testicular self-examination to begin routinely doing so?	**Transparency master** TM 76-1 Diagnostic tests for the male reproductive system **Internet resources** CancerNet: Prostate Cancer http://cancernet.nci.nih.gov/wyntk_pubs/prostate.htm Urology Forum: Erectile Dysfunction http://www.urologychannel.com/erectiledysfunction/index.shtml

4. Identify the procedures for prostate cancer screening. 5. Explain the role of hormonal therapy in treating prostate cancer. 6. Describe the options for treating erectile dysfunction. 7. Discuss the cultural considerations related to male reproductive problems. 8. Analyze assessment data to determine priority nursing diagnoses and collaborative problems for a man with testicular cancer. 9. Develop a plan of care for a client with testicular cancer. 10. Formulate a community-based teaching plan for continuing care of clients with testicular cancer. 11. Compare and contrast hydrocele, spermatocele, and varicocele. 12. Discuss issues related to sexuality and body image for a man experiencing male reproductive health problems.	Identify the advantages of leuprolide acetate (Lupron) or goserelin acetate (Zoladex) injections when given once per month versus daily for clients with advanced prostate cancer. How does the nutritional status of a client affect the success of chemotherapy? Compare the four types of prostate surgery and identify the advantages and disadvantages of each. Describe techniques to reduce scrotal swelling. Explain the possible development of hyponatremia after TURP. Compare the physiological and psychological causes of impotency in men. Describe the use of a pain diary in clients with advanced prostate cancer to help them more accurately describe their pain so that they can obtain better overall relief. How can hair loss from chemotherapy be prevented? Explain why B&O suppositories relieve bladder spasm following TURP. Explain why postorchiectomy hot flashes can be treated with clonidine transdermal patches. Explain why the use of alpha adrenergic blocking agents may delay or omit the need for surgery for BPH. **Pairs check (10-15 min)** Demonstrate the management of a continuous bladder irrigation (CBI) and how intake and output for the client with a CBI should be measured. (Have copies of a sample procedure for the nursing management of a CBI available.) **Numbered heads together (7-10 min)** Ask half the group to describe the use of paclitaxel (Taxol) as a chemotherapeutic agent for treatment of ovarian cancer. (See Chapter 75.) The other half should describe the use of the drug ifosfamide (Ifex) for male clients with testicular cancer.	Prostate Enlargement: BPH http://www.thedailyapple.com/target/cs/article/cs/100664.html The Prostate Help Association http://www.pha.u-net.com/ **Community resources** Assign learners to assess the availability of health information and diagnostic screening facilities related to cancer of the male reproductive system in their immediate area. Go on visits with a hospice nurse and participate in care of at least one terminally ill client as a result of a reproductive health problem. Invite a cancer survivor (either testicular or prostate) from a support group to discuss his or her personal experiences with the disease, treatment, and recovery. Have learners visit a local high school and present concepts about TSE to boys in the upper class levels. Enlist the help of the local health department.

Chapter 77: *Interventions for Clients with Sexually Transmitted Diseases*

Learning Outcomes	Learning Activities	Supplemental Resources
After studying this chapter, the student should be able to: 1. Explain how sexually transmitted diseases (STDs) can be prevented. 2. Compare and contrast the stages of syphilis. 3. Prioritize nursing care for the client with syphilis at each stage. 4. Identify the role of drug therapy in managing clients with genital herpes. 5. Discuss the psychosocial effects of having an STD. 6. Develop a teaching plan for clients diagnosed with gonorrhea. 7. Describe the assessment findings that are typical in clients with *Chlamydia trachomatis* infection. 8. Analyze assessment data to determine common nursing diagnoses for women with pelvic inflammatory disease (PID). 9. Formulate a collaborative plan of care for a client with PID. 10. Develop a community-based teaching plan for clients with PID. 11. Evaluate care for a client with PID. 12. Identify common causes of vaginal infections.	**Think-pair-share (3-5 min)** Compare the types of sexually transmitted diseases. What are some treatments to minimize the discomforts of genital herpes? List street terms for STDs (e.g., the clap and the drip). What are the risk factors for PID? Explain why a lack of vaginal flora leads to recurring bacterial vaginosis. What is the role nurses have in counseling clients with herpes simplex infections? **Concept mapping (10-15 min)** Map ways to break the spread of various sexually transmitted diseases, using the six-step chain on transmission of infection. **Structured controversy (10-15 min)** Should legal restraints concerning transmission of STDs be placed on people known to have these diseases?	**Internet resources** Ask Noah About: Sexually Transmitted Diseases http://www.noah-health.org/english/illness/stds/stds.html i-STD.com http://www.i-std.com/ Urology Forum: STDs http://www.urologychannel.com/std/index.shtml#topofpage Epigee.org: Sexually Transmitted Diseases http://www.epigee.org/guide/stds.html CDC: National Center for HIV, STD, and TB Prevention http://www.cdc.gov/nchstp/od/nchstp.html **Community resources** Attend an interdisciplinary team meeting in a local health department. Invite a local health officer to visit the class and discuss community statistics with respect to STDs. Find out what learners can do to be participative and proactive in helping with the problems. Have a Maternal-Child Clinical Nurse Specialist visit the class and discuss what precautions are taken in hospitals and Birthing Centers to prevent the spread and transmission of STDs in the pregnant population.

TM 74-1

COMPARISON OF SURGICAL PROCEDURES FOR BREAST CANCER

Test	Purpose	Amount of Tissue Removed	Nursing Considerations
Lumpectomy			
Simple mastectomy			
Modified radical mastectomy			
Radical mastectomy			

TM 76-1

DIAGNOSTIC TESTS FOR THE MALE REPRODUCTIVE SYSTEM

Test	Purpose	Client Teaching	Nursing Considerations
Infusion cavernosgraphy			
Nocturnal penile tumescence			
Semen analysis			
Prostatic-specific antigen			
Acid phosphatase			
Alkaline phosphatase			
Alpha-fetoprotein			

CHAPTER 74

Case Study for the Client Having Breast Surgery

A 67-year-old female client presented to her health care provider with a chief complaint of a "lump in my right breast" found when performing breast self-examination (BSE). She was worried that the lump was cancer. Several years ago her mother had a mastectomy for breast cancer. Her mammogram revealed a suspicious lesion. A biopsy of the lesion and axillary lymph nodes confirmed a stage I carcinoma of the right breast with negative lymph nodes. The client's health care provider gave her the option of having a total mastectomy with complete axillary node dissection or breast conservation with lumpectomy, complete axillary node dissection, and radiation therapy. Your client chose breast conserving therapy, and her surgery was performed today. She has returned to your unit for postoperative nursing care. The critical pathway indicates that if her status is stable she will be discharged home tomorrow.

Questions

1. What are the preoperative and postoperative informational needs of this client?

2. How can the nurse support this client in the decision-making process regarding her surgical options?

3. What community resources are available to meet the needs of this client?

4. What are the home care needs of this client?

5. During your home visit your client asks you to do a presentation on breast cancer at the local senior center she attends. What information will you include in your presentation?

CHAPTER 75

Case Study for the Client Having an Abdominal Hysterectomy

Your client is a 44-year-old white woman, with a diagnosis of squamous cell carcinoma of the cervix, who had a total abdominal hysterectomy and bilateral salpingoophorectomy today. She had an estimated blood loss of 30 mL during surgery. Her vital signs and postoperative status are stable. She is to be transferred to your unit for postoperative nursing care.

Questions

1. What initial postoperative assessments should the nurse perform?

2. What are the possible nursing diagnoses for the client who has just had a TAH-BSO?

3. What information should be included in this client's discharge teaching plan?

CHAPTER 77

Case Study for the Client with a Sexually Transmitted Disease

A 22-year-old married female client presents with low abdominal discomfort, dysuria, and menstrual irregularities for 1 month. Her history is noteworthy for episodes of sexually transmitted diseases (gonorrhea, chlamydia, herpes). She seems nervous and distracted during the visit. Your client has been diagnosed with PID and must be admitted to the hospital for intravenous antibiotics. She begins to cry.

Questions

1. What other critical client history questions should you ask?

2. What other physical assessment and laboratory data should you obtain?

3. What assessments/interventions should be completed first?

4. What assessments/interventions should be completed in 24 to 48 hours?

Appendix A

Teaching learners how to develop a nursing process map can be an exciting and stimulating exercise. Clinical postconference time can be used to great advantage for this exercise because (1) group process makes the learning exercise interesting and nonthreatening and (2) the immediacy of clinical experience sharpens learner perceptions of the process.

Assemble learners in a room with a chalkboard or bring in flip chart with paper. If possible, have different colored chalk or marker pens available. For the session, the instructor may choose to do the recording or may ask a learner to volunteer to do the writing.

Student Volunteer Information

Client: 89 y.o. white male, 188 pounds

Chief complaint: shortness of breath for 1 week, pressure in chest

Admitting diagnosis: Congestive heart failure

Past medical history: Congestive heart failure, coronary artery disease, hypertension, coronary artery bypass 8 years ago, prostate surgery 10 years ago

Admission vital signs: T = 97.0° F, P = 80, R = 24, BP = 112/72, Weight = 188 pounds

Laboratory data		*Medications*
Cholesterol level	146	Diagoxin 0.25 mg/day PO
Glucose value	95	Potassium chloride 10 mEq/day PO
Hemoglobin level	38.5	Alprazolam 0.25 mg/HS PO
Hematocrit level	12.3	Quinapril 10 mg/day PO
Platelet count	98,000	Aspirin 81 mg/day PO
Potassium level	3.8	Isosorbide 10 mg/TID PO
Red blood cell count	4.17×10^6	Heparin 5000 U/BID SQ
Sodium value	142	Acetaminophen 650 mg/BID PO
White blood cell count	6.65×10^3	Magnesium hydroxide 30 cc/HS PRN PO
Digoxin levels	0.5	

Physical Examination

Skin pink and dry	egophony throughout lung fields
Nail beds pink, brisk capillary refill	shortness of breath with exertion
Oriented to time, place, and person	dyspnea with exertion
Responds to questions appropriately	crackles at the lung bases bilaterally
Current VS—P = 89, R = 20, BP = 120/67	tires easily
S_3 heart sound	voiding clear, yellow urine 250-400-375 mL per shift
1-cm jugular venous distention	

STEP 1

Ask a volunteer to identify his or her client's information as follows:

A. Identify the client's priority problem or condition, which may be either a medical diagnosis such as congestive heart failure or a pathologic condition such as cystitis.
B. Instruct the recorder to draw the priority problem in the center of the chalkboard.
C. Have the presenter identify the rest of the client's pertinent conditions. It may be helpful to use a symbol for the body system involved.
D. Instruct the recorder to place the rest of the conditions or problems around the priority problem. Ask the recorder to try to put cardiovascular problems in the same general area, respiratory problems in another area, etc.

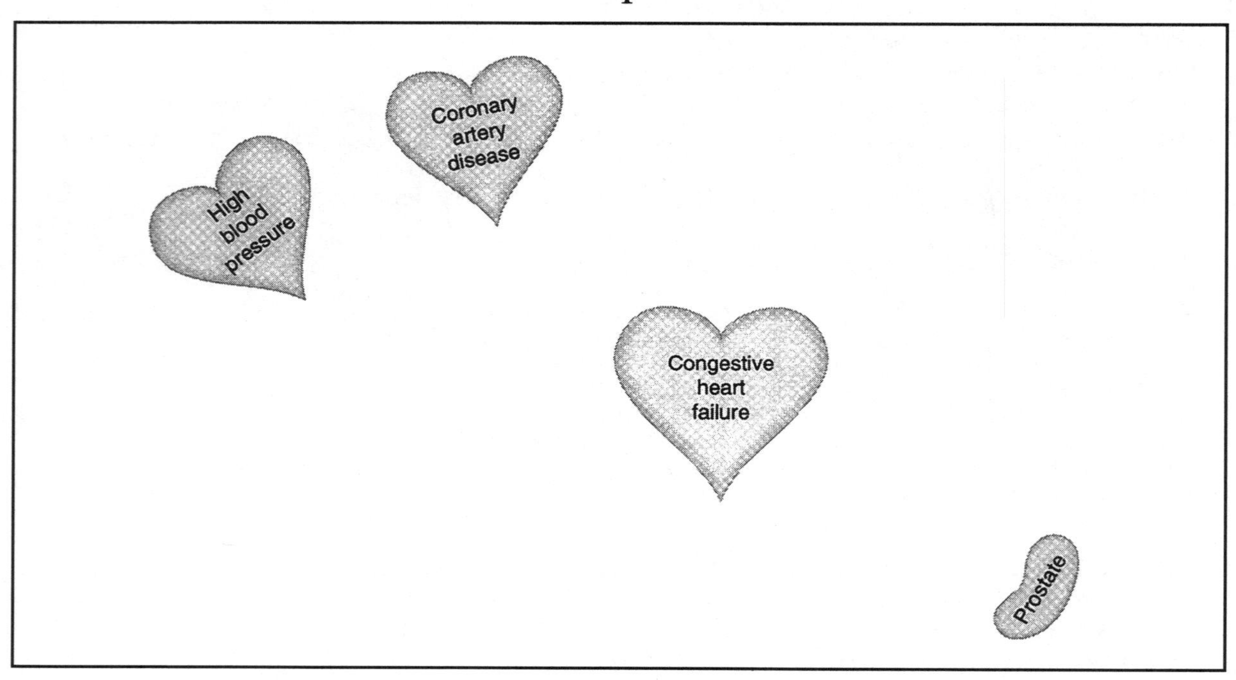

STEP 2

Ask the volunteer presenter to identify the clinical manifestations that their client demonstrated.

A. The learner may need help with some of the associations. Labortory studies, physical examination findings, client interview information, diagnostic tests, and consultation information from other health care professionals may be used. Include psychosocial, developmental, and spiritual responses as appropriate.

Ask the recorder to place the data next to the identified problems in a different colored chalk or marker.

Step 2

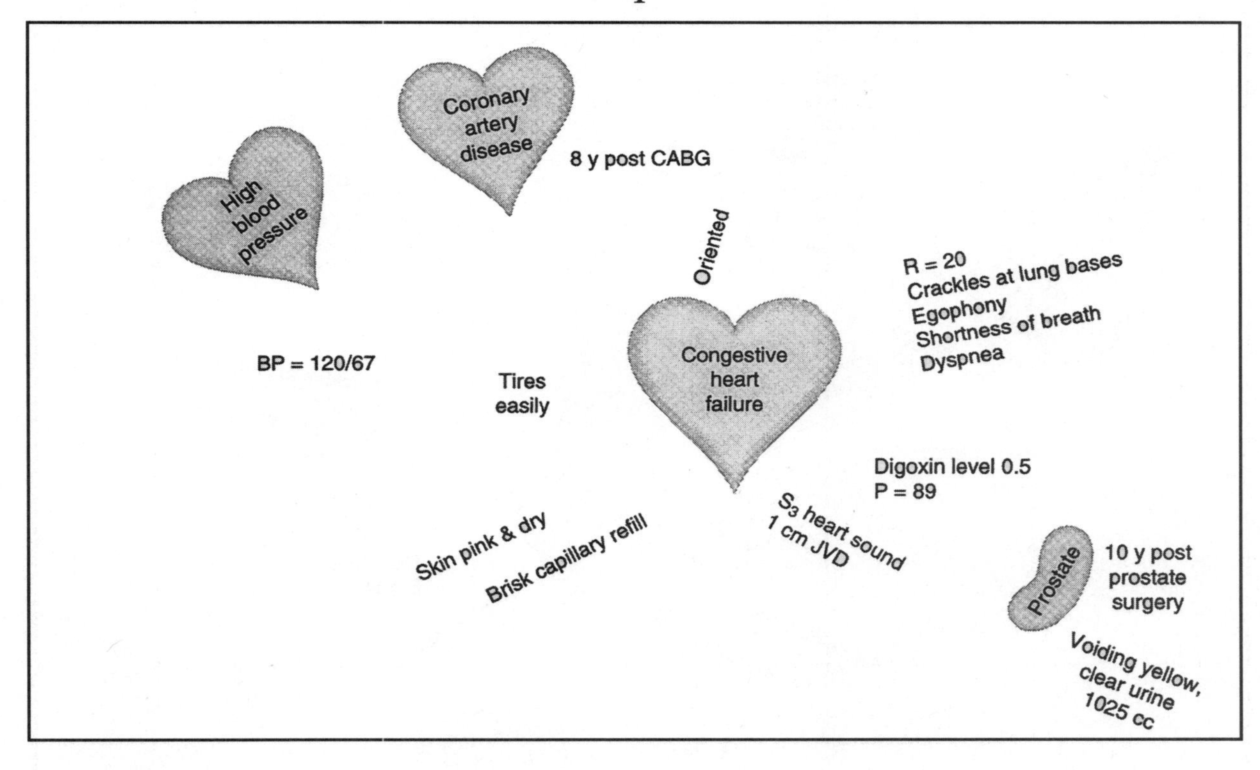

STEP 3

Ask the volunteer presenter to identify the treatment for each of the conditions identified.

A. Medications, oxygen, and other physical treatments may be used. Medical and nursing interventions should be identified.

Ask the recorder to place the data next to the identified problems in a different colored chalk or marker.

Step 3

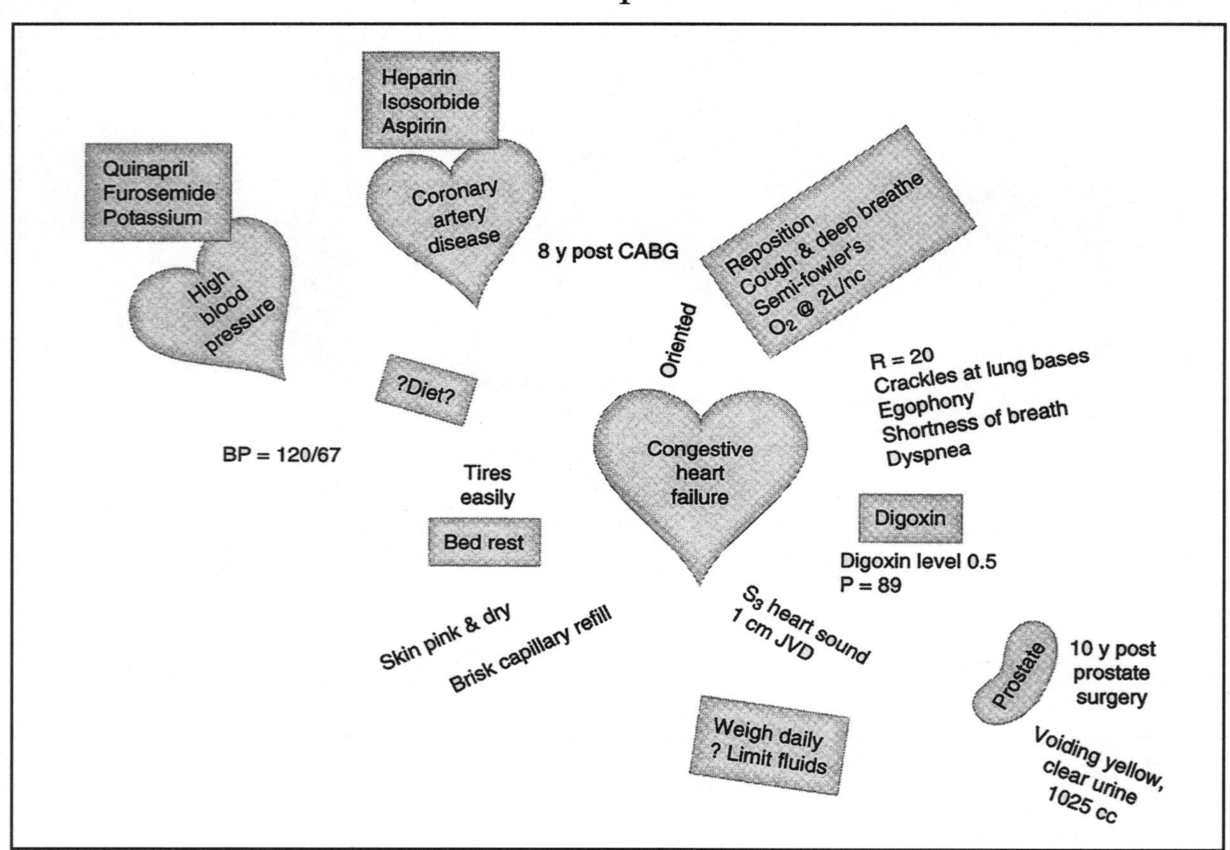

STEP 4

Ask the group as a whole to:

A. Identify the associations and links among the conditons, clinical manifestations, and treatments for the client.

B. Ask the recorder to use a fourth colored chalk or marker to draw arrows indicating associations as the group identifies them.

Step 4

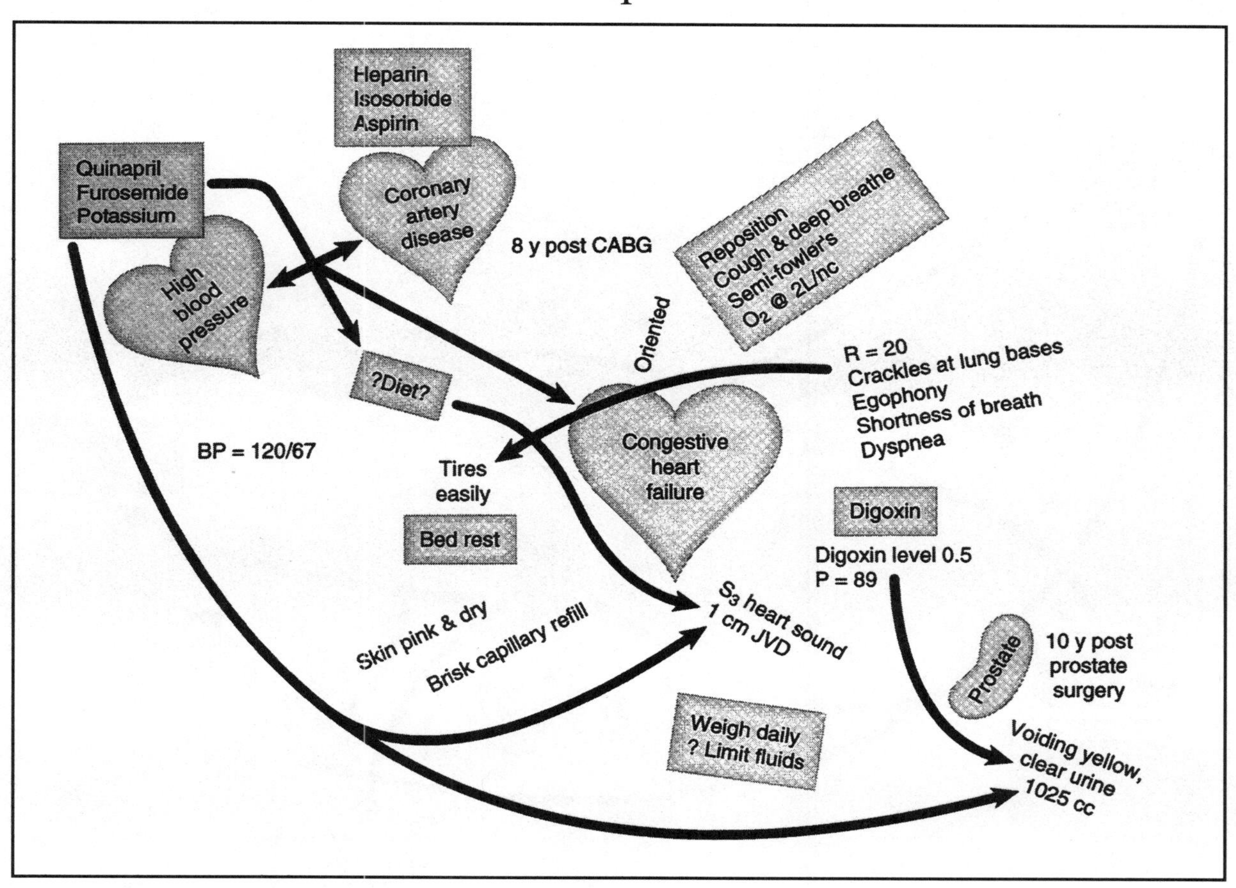

STEP 5

As learners begin to examine the interrelationships, help them to identify appropriate nursing diagnoses, interventions, rationales, and evaluations.

Step 5

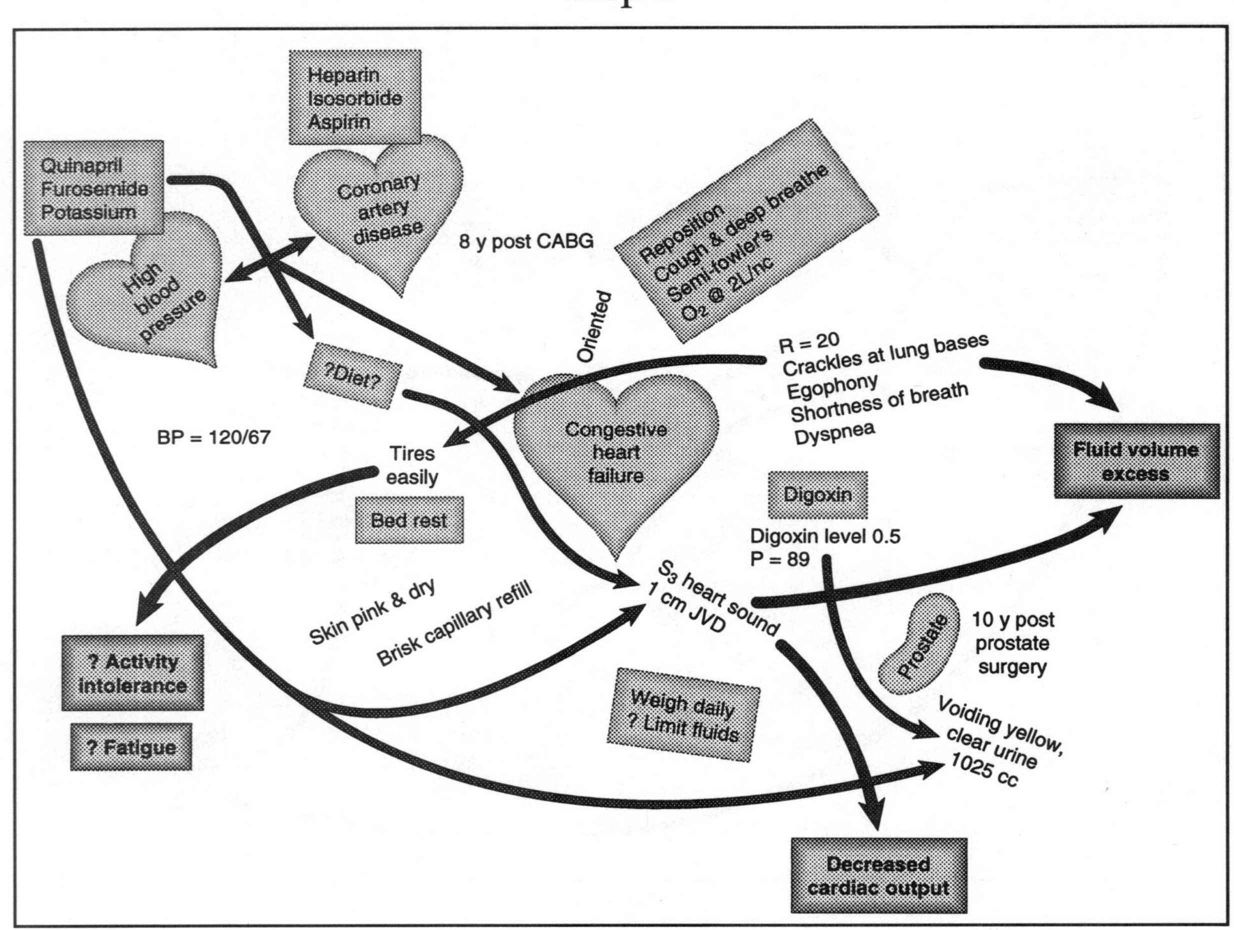

Appendix B

OPEN-BOOK INDEPENDENT LEARNING GUIDE: CARE OF CLIENTS WITH PAIN (Chapter 7)

1. Discuss the incidence and significance of the symptom of pain. What is meant by the description of pain as the "fifth vital sign"? Use at least three definitions of pain in your answer, including your own personal definition. (See textbook pp 61-62.)
2. Describe Gate Control Theory, diagramming the pathway of a painful stimulus. Compare and contrast the different fibers that transmit stimuli. (See textbook pp 62-63.)
3. What are the differences between somatic, visceral, and neuropathic pain? (See textbook pp 63-64.)
4. What is meant by the "subjectivity of pain"? How do the concepts of "pain threshold" and "pain tolerance" influence an individual's perception of pain? (See textbook pp 63-64.)
5. Discuss some of the variables that influence how pain is perceived; for example, age, gender, personality, and cultural background. How might these variables also influence a nurse caring for a client in pain? (See textbook pp 64-66.)
6. Compare and contrast the differences between acute and chronic pain. (See textbook pp 66-69.)
7. How should nursing interventions for the client with chronic nonmalignant pain differ from those for the client with chronic malignant pain? (See textbook pp 67-69.)
8. Describe the elements included in the assessment of a client with pain. How does the nurse modify the assessment when the client is an older adult? (See textbook pp 69-73.)
9. Differentiate between localized pain, projected pain, radiating pain, and referred pain and how they are subjectively described. (See textbook p 70.) Use a pain scale (textbook p 72) and document an assessment on a client experiencing pain.
10. List some appropriate nursing diagnoses or collaborative problems for the client in pain. Write realistic, measurable, time-referenced, expected outcomes for the client. (See textbook pp 73-74, 80.)
11. What are the nursing responsibilities involved in administering opioid analgesics to clients for pain relief? What are some important learning needs for clients receiving them—for example, a client being discharged with a PCA pump? (See textbook pp 74-78, 81-86, 89-90.)
12. What are some additional methods of pain control, both traditional and nontraditional? (See textbook pp 78-80, 86-88.)
13. Discuss some of the ways that nurses should be involved in monitoring pain as a quality improvement (QI) outcome. (See textbook pp 90-92.)

OPEN-BOOK INDEPENDENT LEARNING GUIDE: CARE OF CLIENTS WITH POSTOPERATIVE NEEDS (Chapter 19)

1. What is the general purpose of the postanesthesia care unit (PACU)? (See textbook p 285.)
2. What factors affect postoperative fluid and electrolyte balance? (See textbook p 289.)
3. What are the signs and symptoms of a paralytic ileus? (See textbook p 290.)

4. What is the difference between wound evisceration and dehiscence? What nursing interventions are indicated for each? (See textbook pp 291, 296.)
5. What are the signs and symptoms of an infected postoperative wound? (See textbook p 291.)
6. What is the difference between sanguineous and serous drainage? When should each occur in the postoperative process? (See textbook p 291.)
7. What is the purpose of a surgical drain? What nursing care is involved in caring for the client with a drain? (See textbook pp 291, 292.)
8. Why is Potential for Hypoxemia an appropriate nursing diagnosis in the early postoperative period? What interventions would the nurse anticipate in caring for a client with this nursing diagnosis? (See textbook pp 293-294, 300.)
9. What type of diet would support tissue and wound healing in the postoperative client? (See textbook p 300.)
10. What factors influence when a postoperative client can resume any presurgical activities or work requirements? (See textbook pp 300-301.)

OPEN-BOOK INDEPENDENT LEARNING GUIDE: CARE OF CLIENTS WITH DEGENERATIVE JOINT DISEASE OR RHEUMATOID ARTHRITIS (Chapter 21)

1. What factors contribute to the development of DJD? (See textbook pp 328-329.) Of RA? (See textbook pp 343-344.)
2. What is the relationship between the pathophysiologic changes that occur in the joint of the client with DJD and joint pain? (See textbook pp 328-330.)
3. Why is weight loss a key factor in DJD? (See textbook p 335.)
4. What is the primary contraindication to total joint replacement surgery? (See textbook p 335.)
5. What factors should be included in the preoperative teaching for clients undergoing total joint replacement such as a hip or knee? (See textbook pp 335, 340.)
6. What postoperative nursing interventions are specific to total joint replacement? (See textbook pp 337-341.)
7. What is the function of Lovenox in the joint replacement clients? (See textbook p 339.)
8. What is the etiology of RA? (See textbook p 343.)
9. What factors lead to joint deformity in the client with RA? (See textbook pp 344-346.)
10. What psychologic concerns do clients with RA encounter, and how can the nurse plan to intervene with these needs before they become problematic? (See textbook p 346.)
11. What is the purpose of an antinuclear antibody test? (See textbook p 346.)
12. What are the disadvantages of gold salts in the treatment of RA? (See textbook pp 349-350.)
13. How can the nurse assist the client with RA to manage fatigue? (See textbook p 351.)

OPEN-BOOK INDEPENDENT LEARNING GUIDE: CARE OF CLIENTS WITH COPD/ASTHMA (Chapter 30)

1. What are the pathophysiologic differences between asthma, chronic bronchitis, and pulmonary emphysema? (See textbook pp 529-531.)
2. What is the primary etiology of bronchospasm? (See textbook p 530.)
3. What are the effects of cigarette smoking on lung tissues? (See textbook pp 539-540.)
4. What medical and nursing interventions are required for the client experiencing status asthmaticus? (See textbook p 538.)
5. What is the relationship between lung disease and cardiac failure? (See textbook p 540.)
6. What role does polycythemia have in COPD? (See textbook p 543.)
7. What nursing interventions are involved in the dietary needs of the client with COPD? (See textbook p 550.)
8. What modifications should be made in activities of daily living to promote independence and energy reserve in the client with COPD? (See textbook p 547.)
9. Describe the goals of lung reduction surgery. Describe the postoperative care of clients undergoing this procedure. (See textbook p 546.)
10. What are the home care needs for clients with COPD? (See textbook p 551.)

OPEN-BOOK INDEPENDENT LEARNING GUIDE: CARE OF CLIENTS WITH LUNG CANCER (Chapter 30)

1. Why is the long-term survival rate for lung cancer poor? (See textbook pp 558-559.)
2. How does metastasis from lung cancer occur? (See textbook pp 559-560.)
3. What changes in breath sounds would you expect to hear in a person with lung cancer? (See textbook pp 561-562.)
4. What is the nursing care involved for the client receiving radiation therapy in the treatment of lung cancer? (See textbook p 563.)
5. What is the purpose of and postoperative nursing care involved for the client undergoing wedge resection for lung cancer? (See textbook pp 563-568.)
6. Describe the differences between a one-, two-, and three-bottle chest drainage system and a Pleur-Evac. (See textbook pp 564-568.)
7. What does continuous bubbling in the water seal chamber indicate? What, if any, nursing interventions are indicated? (See textbook p 568.)
8. Describe the positioning involved in the postoperative period for the client with a pnemonectomy. (See textbook p 568.)
9. What signs indicate a thoracentesis may be necessary? (See textbook pp 568-569.)
10. How is dyspnea managed in the client with lung cancer? (See textbook p 569.)

OPEN-BOOK INDEPENDENT LEARNING GUIDE: CARE OF CLIENTS WITH PNEUMONIA (Chapter 31)

1. What clients are at highest risk for developing or contracting pneumonia? (See textbook pp 577-578.)
2. What are the clinical manifestations of pneumonia? (See textbook pp 577-580.)
3. Why might blood cultures be performed on the client with pneumonia? (See textbook p 580.)
4. What is the difference between atelectasis and empyema? (See textbook p 577.)
5. What is incentive spirometry? What teaching principles are involved in instructing a client to perform incentive spirometry? (See textbook p 581.)
6. Why is the client with pneumonia "at risk" for sepsis? (See textbook p 580.)
7. What would the nurse expect to hear in the client with pneumonia who has consolidation? (See textbook p 577.)
8. What should be included in discharge teaching for the client with pneumonia? (See textbook pp 582-583.)

OPEN-BOOK INDEPENDENT LEARNING GUIDE: CARE OF CLIENTS WITH CONGESTIVE HEART FAILURE (Chapter 35)

1. What compensatory mechanisms does the body employ when cardiac output is insufficient to meet body demands? How do each of these increase the heart's output? (See textbook pp 698-699.)
2. What is the difference between preload and afterload? What factors decrease or increase either preload or afterload? (See textbook p 699.)
3. What is the difference between low-output syndrome and high-output syndrome? (See textbook pp 699-700.)
4. What is the pathophysiology behind the development of paroxysmal nocturnal dyspnea? (See textbook p 702.)
5. Why is weight gain the most reliable indicator of fluid gain or loss? (See textbook p 702.)
6. What is the difference between information gained from an ECG and that gained from an echocardiogram? (See textbook p 703.)
7. What nursing interventions and strategies are involved in caring for the client with fluid volume restriction? (See textbook p 707.)
8. What are the cardiac and non-cardiac signs of toxicity of digitalis preparations? (See textbook p 708.)
9. What are the signs of pulmonary edema? How is pulmonary edema related to heart failure? (See textbook p 709.)
10. What community-based resources are available for home care for the client with heart failure? (See textbook pp 710-711.)
11. What symptoms are indicative of worsening heart failure requiring hospital readmisson? (See textbook p 710.)

OPEN-BOOK INDEPENDENT LEARNING GUIDE: CARE OF CLIENTS WITH PERIPHERAL VASCULAR DISEASE (Chapter 36)

1. What is the etiology of peripheral arterial disease? (See textbook p 743.)
2. What is the difference between inflow disease and outflow disease? (See textbook p 744.)
3. Compare and contrast arterial ulcers, diabetic ulcers, and venous stasis ulcers. (See textbook p 745.)
4. What is plethysmography, and what is its usefulness in vascular disease? (See textbook p 746.)
5. What effect does a colder environment have on peripheral vascular disease clients? (See textbook p 748.)
6. Why are antiplatelet agents effective in the treatment of peripheral arterial disease? (See textbook p 747.)
7. What is percutaneous transluminal angioplasty? What outcome would the nurse expect for the client with PVD? (See textbook p 747.)
8. What is the difference between arthrectomy and angioplasty? (See textbook p 747.)
9. What are the signs and symptoms of graft occlusion in the client who has undergone an axillofemoral bypass? (See textbook pp 749-750.)
10. What is the treatment of acute arterial occlusion? Should surgery be necessary, what nursing interventions are involved postoperatively? (See textbook pp 740-751.)

OPEN-BOOK INDEPENDENT LEARNING GUIDE: CARE OF CLIENTS WITH HYPERTENSION (Chapter 36)

1. What is the role of the baroreceptors in hypertension? (See textbook pp 733-734.)
2. What is the role of the renin-angiotensin-aldosterone system in the development of hypertension? (See textbook pp 734-735.)
3. What retinal changes are observed in the client with hypertension? (See textbook p 736.)
4. Why is compliance a problem in the client with hypertension? (See textbook p 736.)
5. What dietary modifications would the nurse expect for the client with hypertension? (See textbook pp 737-738.)
6. Differentiate between the three types of diuretics used in the treatment of hypertension. (See textbook pp 739-740.)
7. What are common side effects of beta-blockers? (See textbook pp 740-741.)
8. What is the difference in regard to drug actions between angiotensin-converting enzyme inhibitors and angitension II receptor antagonists? (See textbook p 741.)
9. Why is the older client at risk for postural hypotension? (See textbook p 741.)
10. What community-based resources are available for the client with hypertension? (See textbook p 742.)
11. Why is weight reduction useful in the client with hypertension? (See textbook pp 742-743.)

OPEN-BOOK INDEPENDENT LEARNING GUIDE: CARE OF CLIENTS WITH A MYOCARDIAL INFARCTION (Chapter 38)

1. What is the relationship between coronary artery disease and myocardial infarction (MI)? (See textbook p 790.)
2. What are the modifiable and non-modifiable risk factors for coronary artery disease and MI? (See textbook p 792.)
3. What is the relationship between angina pectoris and MI? (See textbook pp 793-794.)
4. What serum markers are most indicative of myocardial damage? (See textbook p 795.)
5. Why is ST segment elevation in the ECG often indicative of myocardial damage? (See textbook p 795.)
6. What are the signs and symptoms of MI? (See textbook pp 793-795.)
7. Why is it possible for clients to have vastly different signs and symptoms of MI? (See textbook pp 793-795.)
8. What are the critical facts involved when teaching the client how to take nitroglycerine for relief of chest pain? (See textbook p 795.)
9. What does it mean to titrate morphine for chest pain relief? (See textbook p 795.)
10. What are the parameters for possible complications of the administration of thrombolytics to restore myocardial blood flow? (See textbook pp 798-800.)
11. What are the indications and goals for intra-aortic balloon pumping? (See textbook p 804.)
12. What nursing interventions are involved in the treatment of dysrhythmias? (See textbook p 803.)
13. What is the expected outcome of percutaneous transluminal angioplasty (PTCA)? What sensations might the client experience during PTCA? What nursing care is involved post-PTCA? (See textbook pp 804-806.)

OPEN-BOOK INDEPENDENT LEARNING GUIDE: CARE OF CLIENTS WITH ANEMIA (Chapter 40)

1. Discuss the incidence and the significance of anemia. What is meant by the description of anemia as a "clinical sign rather than a diagnosis"? Describe at least three types and causes of anemia in your answer. Why are the effects of different anemias and the nursing care for clients with those anemias all similar? (See textbook pp 836-837.)
2. Describe sickle cell disease, including its manifestations, incidence, and cultural considerations. What are some factors that influence the development of crises in this disease? What nursing interventions can help reduce the number of chronic long-term manifestations (e.g., sepsis and multiple organ dysfunction)? (See textbook 837-841.)
3. Compare and contrast glucose-6-phosphate dehydrogenase (G6PD) deficiency anemia and immunohemolytic anemia. What teaching could the nurse to provide help in the prevention of exacerbations in clients with these conditions? (See textbook pp 841-842.)
4. What are the differences between anemias caused by hemolytic problems and those caused by a decrease in red blood cell (RBC) production? (See textbook p 842.)
5. Discuss some of the differences between the care of a client with iron deficiency anemia and the client with vitamin B_{12} deficiency anemia. In particular, how would the recommended diet for each vary? What special considerations about vitamin B_{12} injections are necessary for the nurse who is administering them and the client who is receiving them? (See textbook pp 842-844.)

6. Compare and contrast the differences between folic acid deficiency anemia and aplastic anemia. (See textbook p 844.)
7. What special considerations should be made for certain populations who are more susceptible to anemia (e.g., older adults, women during their childbearing years, and clients with poor dietary intake)? (See textbook p 842-843.)
8. Describe the indications for varying types of transfusions: packed RBCs, washed RBCs, plasma, platelets, etc. (See textbook p 842.) What nursing considerations are important in caring for a client who is receiving a transfusion of a blood product? (See textbook pp 862-867.)
9. What are some cultural considerations when caring for a client who needs to receive blood or blood products? (See textbook p 865.)
10. List the types of transfusion reactions, describe the signs and symptoms and the appropriate nursing interventions for each. (See textbook pp 866-867.)
11. Why are many clients encouraged to donate their own blood prior to surgery? What is this type of transfusion called and how is it accomplished? What teaching is important for the client? (See textbook p 867.)

OPEN-BOOK INDEPENDENT LEARNING GUIDE: CARE OF CLIENTS WITH DEMENTIA (Chapter 42)

1. What are the characteristics of Alzheimer's disease (AD)? (See textbook pp 913-916.)
2. What structural and chemical changes occur in the brain of the client with AD? (See textbook p 913.)
3. Compare and contrast the mental changes involved in AD with those of Parkinson's disease. (See textbook pp 909-910, 914-916.)
4. What data can the nurse expect to obtain from the Mini-Mental State Exam (MMSE), and in what ways might nursing intervention need to be adjusted based upon the results of the MMSE? (See textbook p 915.)
5. What changes can the nurse make in the environment of a client with AD to promote greater self-care? (See textbook p 918.)
6. When would psychotropic drugs be considered an option in the treatment plan for a client with AD? (See textbook p 919.)
7. What nursing interventions would help promote safety in a client with AD who is restless or has wandering behavior? (See textbook p 920.)
8. What nursing interventions would help minimize agitation in the client with AD? (See textbook p 920.)
9. What nursing interventions can assist families or caregivers in coping with the strain of providing 24-hour-per-day care for the client with AD? (See textbook p 921.)
10. What community resources are available for the family of the client with AD in regard to respite care? What suggestions regarding activities of daily living needs and home safety concerns could the nurse make to the family of the client with AD? (See textbook pp 920-921.)

OPEN-BOOK INDEPENDENT LEARNING GUIDE: CARE OF CLIENTS WITH STROKE (Chapter 45)

1. What is the difference between an ischemic stroke, a hemorrhagic stroke, and a thrombolytic stroke in regard to incidence, pathophysiology, and signs and symptoms? (See textbook pp 973-976.)

2. What is the difference between a transient ischemic attack (TIA), a reversible ischemic neurologic deficit (RIND), and a stroke? (See textbook p 975.)
3. How might an arteriovenous malformation lead to the development of a stroke? (See textbook p 976.)
4. What are the primary motor signs and symptoms of a stroke? (See textbook p 980.)
5. Why does a stroke occurring in the left hemisphere present with left-sided motor symptoms? (See textbook pp 977, 980.)
6. What are the primary visual changes associated with a stroke? (See textbook p 981.)
7. What is the relationship between hypoxia and increased intracranial pressure (ICP)? (See textbook p 983.)
8. What interventions help decrease the risk in increased ICP? (See textbook pp 983-984.)
9. What is the difference between expressive and receptive aphasia? (See textbook pp 977, 986-987.)
10. What interventions facilitate communication with clients experiencing receptive or expressive aphasia? (See textbook p 987.)
11. What safety measures should the nurse use in feeding the client with swallowing difficulties? (See textbook p 987.)
12. What community resources are available to assist the family of the client with a stroke? (See textbook pp 988-989.)

OPEN-BOOK INDEPENDENT LEARNING GUIDE: CARE OF CLIENTS WITH FRACTURES (Chapter 52)

1. What is the difference between an open fracture and a closed fracture? Which type is most likely to become infected, and why? (See textbook pp 1125, 1129.)
2. Describe at least three potentially life-threatening complications related to fractures. What collaborative management, including monitoring, is needed to prevent or detect these complications? (See textbook pp 1127-1129, 1132-1133.)
3. What is the difference between closed and open reduction of fractures? (See textbook pp 1133-1140.)
4. What nursing interventions are required for a client who has a cast? (See textbook pp 1133-1136.)
5. What is the difference between skin and skeletal traction? What nursing interventions are required for clients in traction? (See textbook pp 1136-1137.)
6. What other members of the interdisciplinary team may be involved in the care of a client with a fracture, and why? (See textbook pp 1140-1141.)
7. How is pain managed for a client who has experienced a fracture? (See textbook p 1139.)
8. What is the primary cause of hip fractures in older adults? How can they be prevented? (See textbook pp 1142-1143.)
9. What special body positioning is needed postoperatively for the older adult who has had an ORIF of the hip? Why is this position necessary? (See textbook p 1145.)
10. What community-based care should be provided for a client who has experienced a fracture? (See textbook pp 1141-1142.)

OPEN-BOOK INDEPENDENT LEARNING GUIDE: CARE OF CLIENTS WITH PEPTIC ULCER DISEASE (PUD) (Chapter 56)

1. Discuss the incidence and significance of peptic ulcers. Differentiate between the characteristics of gastric, duodenal, and stress ulcers. (See textbook pp 1218-1220.)
2. What are the categories and types of pharmacologic agents that are commonly used to treat peptic ulcer disease (PUD)? (See Chart 56-3 and textbook pp 1218-1219.)
3. What are the most common complications resulting from PUD? Describe four of these complications—chart the incidence, etiology, signs, and symptoms of each complication. (See textbook 1220-1221.)
4. What is the relationship between PUD and the use of nonsteroidal anti-inflammatory drugs (NSAIDs)? Describe the course of PUD in clients who are receiving NSAIDs. (See textbook p 1221.)
5. What is the relationship between bacterial *Helicobacter pylori* and PUD? How is this bacteria transmitted? What additional substances and pharmacologic agents often contribute to the development of PUD? (See textbook p 1221-1222.)
6. Compose a questionnaire that asks appropriate questions about the history of a client with suspected PUD. What is included? What are the factors placing the client at risk for PUD? (See textbook p 1222.)
7. What special considerations should be made for certain populations who are more susceptible to PUD for (e.g., older adults)? (See textbook p 1222.)
8. Describe the physical assessment for a client with PUD. What are the typical subjective data? Objective data? Differentiate between the symptom of pain caused by a gastric ulcer and a duodenal ulcer. (See textbook pp 1222-1223.)
9. Discuss typical assessments in a client with PUD, taking into account physical, psychologic, laboratory, radiologic, and other diagnostic findings. (See textbook pp 1222-1224.)
10. Establish a nursing diagnosis for a client with PUD. Write a measurable, realistic, time-oriented outcome and list nursing interventions to achieve the desired outcome. (See textbook p 1224.)
11. Make a chart listing the most frequently used pharamacologic agents currently being used to treat PUD. Include categories, costs, actions, and effectiveness, as well as each drug's effects on older adults with the disease. (See textbook pp 1224-1226.)
12. Compare and contrast various methods of treating the fluid deficit problem caused by the bleeding of PUD. Differentiate between nonsurgical and surgical managements/interventions. (See textbook pp 1226-1232.)
13. Describe the placement and care of nasogastric tubes. (See textbook pp 1227-1230.)
14. Discuss the surgical treatments of PUD and the care required for the client postoperatively. Include considerations for management in the home environment after discharge. (See textbook pp 1228-1234.)

OPEN-BOOK INDEPENDENT LEARNING GUIDE: CARE OF CLIENTS WITH CHRONIC INFLAMMATORY BOWEL DISEASE (IBD) (Chapter 58)

1. Discuss the incidence and significance of chronic inflammatory bowel disease (IBD). Differentiate between the characteristics of the two major groups of chronic IBDs: ulcerative colitis and Crohn's disease. (See textbook 1274-1276, 1283-1285.)
2. What are the most common complications that accompany ulcerative colitis? (See Chart 58-3 and textbook 1275.)

3. Describe the components of an assessment of a client with ulcerative colitis, paying particular attention to psychologic as well as physical parameters. (See textbook pp 1275-1276.)
4. Compile a list of plausible nursing diagnoses or collaborative problems for a client with ulcerative colitis. Establish realistic, measurable, time-referenced expected outcomes based on these diagnoses. (See textbook p 1276.)
5. Discuss methods and interventions of nonsurgical management (with emphasis on diet and drug treatments) of some of the signs and symptoms of ulcerative colitis. (See textbook pp 1276-1278.)
6. Compose a teaching aid for a client recently diagnosed with ulcerative colitis who is being discharged home. Include dietary, pharmacologic and lifestyle needs and changes. (See textbook pp 1276-1278.)
7. Discuss the surgical management of a client with ulcerative colitis, including postoperative care, pain management, and monitoring for complications. What percentage of clients with the disease will require surgery? (See textbook pp 1279-1282.)
8. Describe the education necessary for a client who has recently had an ileostomy performed. (See textbook pp 1280-1283.)
9. Discuss typical assessments in a client with Crohn's disease, taking into account physical, psychologic, laboratory, radiologic, and other diagnostic findings. (See textbook pp 1283-1285.)
10. Establish a nursing diagnosis for a client with Crohn's disease. Write a measurable, realistic, time-oriented outcome, and list nursing interventions to achieve the desired outcome. (See textbook pp 1283-1287.)
11. What are some considerations (i.e., costs, teaching, home care) in planning long-term care for the client with Crohn's disease? (See textbook p 1287.)

OPEN-BOOK INDEPENDENT LEARNING GUIDE: CARE OF CLIENTS WITH CIRRHOSIS (Chapter 59)

1. Discuss the incidence, etiology, and significance of cirrhosis. Differentiate among the four major types of cirrhosis: Laënnec's (alcoholic), postnecrotic, biliary, and cardiac. (See textbook pp 1298-1299, 1301.)
2. What are the most common complications that accompany cirrhosis? Make a chart that describes the causes and results of each. (See textbook pp 1299-1301.)
3. Describe an assessment of a client with end-stage cirrhosis. Discuss nursing interventions for identified problems. (See textbook p 1300 and chart on p 1306.)
4. What does the physical assessment of a client with undiagnosed early stage cirrhosis entail? (See textbook pp 1301-1302.) As the disease progresses, how do assessment findings change? (See textbook pp 1302-1303.)
5. Discuss significant laboratory, radiologic, and other assessments in a client with cirrhosis (e.g., an EGD). (See textbook pp 1303-1304.)
6. Compile a list of plausible nursing diagnoses for a client with cirrhosis. Establish realistic, measurable, time-referenced outcomes based on these diagnoses. (See pp 1304-1305.)
7. Discuss the nonsurgical management of a client with cirrhosis. What nursing responsibilities are involved in diet and drug therapy, in assisting with paracentesis, and in providing for the client's comfort? (See textbook p 1305.)
8. Which clients with cirrhosis and resulting ascites should have a paracentesis performed, and which are candidates for a surgical shunt? (See textbook pp 1305-1308.)

9. What medical and nursing interventions are necessary for the client with cirrhosis and resulting hemorrhagic problems (coagulation problems, esophageal varices)? (See textbook pp 1308-1311.)
10. What is portal-systemic encephalopathy (PSE), and how does a nurse monitor for it in the client with cirrhosis? What diet and drug teaching should the nurse implement in the client with PSE? (See textbook pp 1311-1312.)
11. Compose a teaching plan for a client recently diagnosed with cirrhosis who is being discharged home. Include dietary, pharmacologic, and lifestyle needs and changes. (See textbook pp 1312-1313.)

OPEN-BOOK INDEPENDENT LEARNING GUIDE: CARE OF CLIENTS WITH PANCREATITIS (Chapter 60)

1. Discuss the incidence, etiology, and significance of pancreatitis. Differentiate between the acute and chronic types of pancreatitis. (See textbook pp 1338-1340, 1345-1346.)
2. What are the four major pathophysiologic processes that accompany pancreatitis? Make a chart that describes the causes and results of each. (See textbook pp 1338-1339.)
3. Describe the history and assessment of a client with acute pancreatitis. Discuss the psychosocial, laboratory, radiographic, and other diagnostic findings expected in a client with acute pancreatitis. (See textbook pp 1340-1342.)
4. Compile a list of plausible nursing diagnoses or collaborative problems for a client with acute pancreatitis. (See textbook p 1342.) Establish realistic, measurable, time-referenced expected outcomes based on these diagnoses. (See textbook pp 1342-1344.)
5. Discuss specific interventions to deal with a major symptom of acute pancreatitis: acute pain. (See textbook pp 1342-1343.)
6. Compose a teaching plan for a client recently diagnosed with acute pancreatitis who is being discharged home. Include dietary, pharmacologic, and lifestyle needs and changes. (See textbook pp 1344-1345.)
7. Describe the history and assessment of a client with chronic pancreatitis. Discuss the psychosocial, laboratory, radiographic, and other diagnostic findings expected in a client with chronic pancreatitis. (See textbook pp 1346-1347.)
8. Discuss methods and interventions of nonsurgical management (with emphasis on diet, enzyme replacement, and drug treatments) of some of the signs and symptoms of chronic pancreatitis. (See textbook p 1347.)
9. Compose a teaching plan for a client with chronic pancreatitis who is being discharged home. Include dietary, pharmacologic, and lifestyle needs and changes. (See textbook p 1348.)
10. What can the nurse teach the client with chronic pancreatitis who wants to prevent exacerbations of the disease? (See textbook p 1348 and Chart 60-8.)

OPEN-BOOK INDEPENDENT LEARNING GUIDE: CARE OF CLIENTS WITH HYPOTHYROIDISM OR HYPERTHYROIDISM (Chapter 64)

1. What role do thyroid hormones play in normal body functioning? (See textbook pp 1423-1424.)
2. What ophthalmic changes are expected in hyperthyroidism? (See textbook pp 1425-1426.)
3. Describe the management of hyperthyroidism by drug therapy and radioactive iodine therapy. What client teaching needs are involved in the client receiving either of these therapies? (See textbook pp 1427-1428.)

4. What nursing interventions are involved in the client post-thyroidectomy? (See textbook pp 1429-1430.)
5. What is the relationship between hypocalcemia and thyroidectomy? (See textbook p 1429.)
6. What are the manifestations of thyroid storm, and what interventions should the nurse be prepared to implement? (See textbook p 1429.)
7. How do the clinical manifestations of hypothyroidism differ from those of hyperthyroidism? (See textbook pp 1431-1432.)
8. What are the clinical manifestations of myxedema? (See textbook p 1434.)
9. Why is hypothyroidism considered a lifelong disease? (See textbook p 1434.)
10. Why should all clients with hypothyroidism wear a MedicAlert bracelet? (See textbook p 1434.)

OPEN-BOOK INDEPENDENT LEARNING GUIDE: CARE OF CLIENTS WITH DIABETES (Chapter 65)

1. What are the functions of insulin? (See textbook pp 1442-1443.)
2. What happens when insulin is absent? What signs and symptoms would you expect to see in client with no natural insulin production? (See textbook p 1443.)
3. What are the chronic complications of diabetes, and how might these be prevented or lessened? (See textbook pp 1444-1445.)
4. What are the primary differences between type I and type II diabetes? (See textbook p 1447.)
5. What does the finding of an elevated glycosylated hemoglobin (HbA_{1c}) mean? (See textbook pp 1450-1451.)
6. Explain the difference in action and effect of oral hypoglycemic agents and insulin. (See textbook pp 1452-1458.)
7. What new insulin injection techniques are available for the client requiring daily insulin injections? (See textbook pp 1460-1461.)
8. Why is accurate self-glucose monitoring essential to the well-being of diabetics? (See textbook p 1462.)
9. What are the nutrition educational needs of the client with diabetes? (See textbook pp 1465-1467.)
10. What is the relationship between nutrition, exercise, and the maintenance of appropriate blood sugar levels in the client with diabetes? (See textbook pp 1467-1469.)
11. What are the risks involved and the success rates of pancreas or islet cell transplantation? (See textbook pp 1469-1470.)
12. What are the preoperative and postoperative needs of the diabetic client who must undergo surgery? (See textbook pp 1471-1472.)
13. What are the integumentary risks for the client with diabetes? What should the diabetic client be taught regarding skin and foot care? (See textbook pp 1472-1473.)
14. What should the diabetic client be taught regarding the management of hypoglycemic episodes? (See textbook pp 1475-1476.)
15. What should the diabetic client be taught regarding the management of ketoacidotic episodes? (See textbook pp 1481-1482.)
16. What is hyperglycemic-hyperosmolar nonketotic syndrome, and how is it managed? (See textbook pp 1483-1484.)

17. What are the many psychosocial needs of the client with diabetes, and how can the nurse assist the client in the maintenance of emotional well-being? (See textbook pp 1485-1486.)

OPEN-BOOK INDEPENDENT LEARNING GUIDE: CARE OF CLIENTS WITH A PRESSURE ULCER (Chapter 67)

1. In which anatomic location do pressure ulcers primarily form? (See textbook p 1519.)
2. What is the relationship between pressure, friction, and shear forces in the development of pressure ulcers? (See textbook p 1519.)
3. What factors are involved in a pressure ulcer prevention program? (See textbook p 1520.)
4. What is the relationship between nutritional status and ulcer formation? (See textbook p 1521.)
5. What is the relationship between incontinence and ulcer formation? (See textbook pp 1521-1522.)
6. What equipment is available for the prevention of pressure ulcers? (See textbook p 1523.)
7. What role does positioning play in the prevention of pressure ulcers? (See textbook p 1523.)
8. What factors are involved in the assessment of pressure ulcer wounds? (See textbook pp 1523-1524.)
9. What is the difference between a hydrophobic and a hydrophilic dressing in the treatment of pressure ulcers? (See textbook p 1527.)
10. What foods will promote tissue healing in the client with pressure ulcers? (See textbook pp 1527-1528.)
11. What surgical interventions are available for the client with pressure ulcers? Describe the nursing care involved. (See textbook pp 1529-1531.)
12. What nursing interventions will assist in the prevention of infection and wound extension in the client with a pressure ulcer? (See textbook p 1531.)

OPEN-BOOK INDEPENDENT LEARNING GUIDE: CARE OF CLIENTS WITH BURNS (Chapter 68)

1. In simple terms, what is the difference between superficial-thickness, partial-thickness, full-thickness, and deep full-thickness burns? (See textbook pp 1556-1559.)
2. What is the difference between fluid shift and fluid remobilization? When do these occur after a burn? What type of fluid resuscitation is involved in burn therapy? (See textbook pp 1559-1560.)
3. What changes are seen in the lungs of the client with a burn inhalation injury? What signs and symptoms will the client exhibit? What nursing interventions are involved in promoting good ventilation status? (See textbook pp 1560-1561.)
4. What is the rule for the calculation of size and depth of burn injury? (See textbook pp 1567-1568.)
5. Why do the caloric needs of the client with burn injury double or triple? (See textbook p 1561.)
6. What is the purpose of an escharotomy and debridement in the burn client? What types of debridement are available in the care of the burned client? (See textbook pp 1572, 1577.)
7. How is pain managed in the burn client? (See textbook pp 1573-1576.)
8. What options are available for skin donation and grafting? (See textbook p 1578.)

9. Why is infection a primary threat to the burn client, and what interventions are used to minimize this risk? (See textbook pp 1579-1580.)
10. What interventions are aimed toward maintaining mobility in the client with burns? (See textbook pp 1582-1583.)
11. What is the nurse's role in dealing with the possible devastating psychologic effects of severe burns? What interventions are involved? (See textbook pp 1583-1584.)
12. What factors are involved in the rehabilitative phase of burn injury? What is the nurse's role during this time? (See textbook p 1584.)

OPEN-BOOK INDEPENDENT LEARNING GUIDE: CARE OF CLIENTS WITH CHRONIC RENAL FAILURE (Chapter 72)

1. What factors lead to the progression of the development of chronic renal failure (CRF)? (See textbook pp 1675-1676.)
2. What role do urea, creatinine, sodium, and potassium play in CRF? (See textbook pp 1676-1677.)
3. What are the symptoms of metabolic acidosis in relation to CRF? (See textbook p 1677.)
4. Why is hypertension a problem for the client with CRF? (See textbook p 1678.)
5. What factors lead to the development of hypertension in CRF? (See textbook p 1678.)
6. Why do CHF and pulmonary edema pose significant risks for the client with CRF? (See textbook p 1678.)
7. Describe the dietary needs of the client with CRF. (See textbook pp 1679, 1682-1683.)
8. What unique integumentary changes occur with CRF? What nursing interventions are involved in assisting clients in coping with these changes? (See textbook p 1681.)
9. What information should the nurse gain from BUN levels and glomerular filtration rates? (See textbook pp 1676-1678.)
10. Describe the role of dialysis (peritoneal and hemodialysis) in the treatment of CRF. Compare and contrast the nursing care needs of both types of dialysis. (See textbook pp 1688-1692, 1693-1696.)
11. What assessments should the nurse make in monitoring the vascular access device of a dialysis patient? What are the most common complications of vascular access devices? (See textbook p 1690.)
12. What psychosocial issues are involved in helping the client with CRF cope with this lifelong disease? (See textbook pp 1701-1702.)
13. Discuss community resources available for clients with CRF and their families. (See textbook p 1702.)

OPEN-BOOK INDEPENDENT LEARNING GUIDE: CARE OF CLIENTS WITH BREAST CANCER (Chapter 74)

1. Discuss the incidence, etiology, risk factors, and significance of breast cancer. (See textbook p 1736.)
2. What is the major pathophysiologic process that accounts for the majority of cases of breast cancer? Diagram this process. Discuss the significance of what is meant by "dimpling." (See textbook p 1736.)
3. Describe the complications of breast cancer as well as the course of the disease. What is the incidence in men, and how does the course of the disease differ? (See textbook pp 1736-1737.)

4. Compile a list of plausible risk factors that contribute to the development of breast cancer. (See textbook pp 1737-1738.) How do the variables of age and culture influence the risk for the development of breast cancer? (See textbook p 1738.)
5. Describe the history taking and multiple assessments in a client with breast cancer. Discuss the psychosocial (including health maintenance practices), laboratory, radiographic, and other diagnostic findings expected in a client with breast cancer. (See textbook p 1738-1740.)
6. Compile a list of plausible nursing diagnoses or collaborative problems for the client with breast cancer. (See textbook pp 1740-1741, 1744-1745.) Establish realistic, measurable, time-referenced expected outcomes based on these diagnoses. (See textbook pp 1741, 1744-1745.)
7. Discuss methods and interventions in treating clients with breast cancer using nonsurgical management techniques (with an emphasis on palliative care and varying treatment modalities). (See textbook pp 1741-1742.)
8. Discuss the surgical management of the client with breast cancer, including preoperative and postoperative care, pain management, and monitoring for complications. What percentage of clients with the disease will require some form of surgery (mastectomy)? (See textbook pp 1742-1744.)
9. Compose a teaching plan for a client with breast cancer who is being discharged home. Include dietary, pharmacologic/further treatment, and lifestyle/psychosocial needs and changes. (See textbook pp 1744, 1746-1749.)
10. What can the nurse tell the client with breast cancer who wants to know more about the possibilities of reconstructive surgery? (See textbook pp 1744-1746 and Table 74-5.)

OPEN-BOOK INDEPENDENT LEARNING GUIDE: CARE OF CLIENTS WITH DYSFUNCTIONAL UTERINE BLEEDING (DUB) AND HYSTERECTOMY (Chapter 76)

1. Discuss the incidence and significance of dysfunctional uterine bleeding (DUB). Differentiate between the characteristics of the causes of this condition and its manifestations. (See textbook p 1756.)
2. What are the most common signs and symptoms that accompany DUB? (See textbook p 1756.)
3. Describe the components of an assessment of a client with DUB, paying attention to the psychologic (stress) as well as physical parameters. (See textbook p 1756.)
4. Compile a list of plausible nursing diagnoses or collaborative problems for a client with DUB. Establish realistic, measurable, time-referenced expected outcomes based on these diagnoses. (See textbook p 1756.)
5. Discuss methods and interventions of nonsurgical management (with emphasis on hormonal therapy) of some of the signs and symptoms of DUB. (See textbook p 1756.)
6. Compose a teaching aid for a client recently diagnosed with DUB. Include dietary, pharmacologic, and lifestyle needs and changes. (See textbook p 1756.)
7. Discuss the surgical management of a client with DUB, beginning with the least invasive (D & C) and progressing to the most complex (hysterectomy). What percentage of clients with the disease will require surgery? (See textbook pp 1756, 1766-1768.)
8. Describe the education necessary for a client who has recently had a hysterectomy performed. (See textbook pp 1768, and Chart 75-9.)
9. Discuss common postoperative complications in a client following hysterectomy. (See textbook pp 1767-1768.)

10. Establish a nursing diagnosis or collaborative problem for an older client who has had a hysterectomy. Write a measurable, realistic, time-oriented expected outcome, and list nursing interventions to achieve the desired outcome. (See textbook pp 1766-1768.)

11. What are some considerations (i.e., costs, teaching, home care) in planning for the discharge of a client who has had a hysterectomy? (See textbook pp 1767-1768.)

Appendix C

Teaching with the Virtual Clinical Excursions Workbook/CD-ROM

VCE Workbook

Virtual Clinical Excursions for Ignatavicius & Workman: *Medical-Surgical Nursing: Critical Thinking for Collaborative Care,* fourth edition, is a *workbook* that sends the student into a virtual hospital setting to learn communication, documentation, assessment, critical thinking, and other essential skills. Through both written and CD-ROM activities, the workbook guides the student to collect information, make decisions, and set priorities within the virtual hospital setting. The student spends a week in a virtual hospital with *five patients*, participating in clinical rotations and examining the patients' data.

The workbook has two CD-ROMs – Disk 1 (Installation) and Disk 2 (Patients' Disk). The student "visits" each of the five patients and accesses and evaluates realistic information resources essential for patient care. Information resources in the virtual hospital include: charts, medication administration records, electronic patient records, video streaming of patient dialogue with nurses, and other related materials. The student also has access to the virtual hospital's Website and an online medical library.

How to Use the VCE Workbook

Virtual Clinical Excursions presents five patients just as a floor presents patients during a clinical rotation. The workbook provides guidance on how to use the nursing process to care for patients in the virtual hospital.

As each patient's condition changes through time in the virtual hospital, the workbook helps the students learn how to reassess and develop new diagnoses, decide on desirable outcomes, select interventions to achieve these outcomes, and evaluate whether the outcomes were achieved.

1. If you teach online, i.e., in a computer lab, you can instruct your students to work independently to complete a lesson and then, in a small group, discuss different approaches and variations. As the group monitor, you can critique and provide input. For example, you can discuss the patient data that should be collected and the priorities that need to be set for collecting these data.
2. You can assign a lesson and have students work independently outside class and then conduct a broad discussion in class, such as might be found in a nursing grand round. You can also divide the class into smaller groups for discussion.
3. You can use the patients in the virtual hospital to lead discussions in a specific subject area. For example, after teaching about cardiovascular disease, you can present a couple of the patients in the virtual hospital (e.g., Carmen Gonzales and Sally Begay) and ask the students to evaluate the patients in the context of what they have learned about cardiovascular disease. This will allow you to examine the translation from "book learning" to development of clinical judgment.
4. The patients in the virtual hospital can be used as a focus for discussion of a clinical scenario both prior to and after a clinical rotation. For example, in a pre-clinical conference, the patients in the virtual hospital can be used to discuss particular approaches to assessing certain kinds of patients. In a post-clinical conference, the patients in the virtual hospital can be used in debriefing to discuss variances discovered in real patients that are not found in the clinical simulations.
5. The patients in the virtual hospital can be used for students who have missed a clinical assignment. You can assign students who missed clinical to work on one or more patients, and then have these students attend a working session in which the simulations and nursing care are discussed in detail. **(Note: This software is *not* a replacement for real clinicals.)**

6. You can use the patients in the virtual hospital to discuss the case mix to which students are exposed during their clinical experiences. For example, students may not get a chance to work with an AIDS patient, so they can work as a class on Ira Bradley, a patient in the virtual hospital. Or, students may not be exposed to various ethnic populations, so they could work as a class to examine the transcultural nursing issues for patients like Carmen Gonzales (Spanish-speaking citizen), Sally Begay (Native American), David Ruskin (African American), or Andrea Wang (Asian American).

The Five Patients

Andrea Wang

Diagnosis: Spinal cord injury

Admission: Andrea Wang, a 20-year-old Asian female, is admitted to the hospital after a diving injury that resulted in a crushed T6 vertebrae and partial transection of the spinal cord.

Hospital Course: She is in spinal shock on admission and has spent 1 week in the ICU prior to being transferred to a medical-surgical unit. The student begins care on day 9 of her hospitalization.

Significant Case Concerns: Andrea Wang's clinical case progresses as expected. Significant identified concerns include weight-loss since admission, autonomic dysreflexia, bowel and bladder retraining, aging parents and family coping issues, lack of a social support network, sexuality and intimacy concerns with her boyfriend, self-image adjustment, and overall rehabilitation plan.

Carmen Gonzales

Diagnoses: Gangrenous leg; diabetes mellitus, type 2; congestive heart failure; osteomyelitis

Admission: Carmen Gonzales, a 56-year-old Hispanic female, is admitted to the hospital with an infected leg that has become gangrenous. She has type 2 diabetes mellitus, as well as congestive heart failure and osteomyelitis complications.

Hospital Course: She is admitted to the hospital on a Sunday. She is taken to the operating room for debridement of her leg wound. Her wound is healing as expected. A fluid overload during the perioperative period has resulted in an exacerbation of her congestive heart failure. The student begins care on day 3 of her hospitalization.

Significant Case Concerns: Carmen Gonzales has several past hospitalizations for her diabetes and related complications. Although she speaks some English, Spanish is her primary language. She lives with her husband, who is retired. They lead a traditional Hispanic lifestyle. Dietary habits are a daily challenge for compliance with her prescribed diabetic diet. Because she is the primary breadwinner in the family, her current hospitalization and complications are a great concern. She has many concerns about her future, finances, and continued medical illnesses.

David Ruskin

Diagnoses: Possible closed head injury; closed fracture right humerus

Admission: David Ruskin, a 31-year-old African-American male, is admitted after a car-bicycle crash. He has a fractured right humerus and a possible closed head injury.

Hospital Course: He is admitted to the hospital on a Sunday and is taken to the operating suite for open reduction and internal fixation of the right humerus. Because of the injury history and early clinical signs, he is monitored carefully for a possible closed head injury. It is identified that he also has bruising of the chest wall and some discomfort with respirations. He continues to have some orientation problems. The student begins care on day 3 of his hospitalization.

Significant Case Concerns: David Ruskin does well postoperatively until the Thursday following admission. His clinical signs and a low-grade fever indicate a possible pulmonary or fat embolus. This must be ruled out. David Ruskin is in an interracial marriage. His wife is pregnant with their first child. During the hospital period, the nurse learns of his concerns related to the pregnancy.

Ira Bradley

Diagnoses: HIV-AIDS; opportunistic respiratory infection; oral fungal infection; malnutrition and wasting

Admission: Ira Bradley, a 43-year-old white male in late-stage HIV infection, is admitted for an opportunistic respiratory infection. He has complications of oral fungal infection, malnutrition, and wasting. There are also numerous complex patient-family psychosocial concerns.

Hospital Course: Ira Bradley's opportunistic respiratory and oral fungal infections respond to therapy during the hospital stay. He has significant nutritional and electrolyte imbalances secondary to his not eating and his body wasting. The case conference that occurs during the hospital stay addresses the multitude of physical, sociocultural, economic, and behavioral concerns. The student begins care on day 3 of his hospitalization.

Significant Case Concerns: Ira Bradley has had significant malnutrition and wasting since his last hospitalization. Eating is difficult for him, and his outlook toward the future is low. Mrs. Bradley is continuously with him, and between them, they present the nurse with the many difficult issues related to HIV, such as isolation from family and friends, sexuality, finances, and overall coping. Mrs. Bradley has difficulty staying employed because of increasing care-giving demands, while the Bradley children are being rejected by their peers because of the stigma of their father's illness.

Sally Begay

Diagnoses: Bacterial lung infection; chronic obstructive pulmonary disease; history of coronary artery disease and hypertension

Admission: Sally Begay, a 58-year-old Native-American female, is admitted to the hospital with the initial diagnosis to rule out *Hantavirus* infection. She also has controlled coronary artery disease (CAD), hypertension, and chronic obstructive pulmonary disease (COPD).

Hospital Course: Because she lives on a reservation and had been working in the barn where mouse droppings were prevalent, it is first thought that she most likely has a *Hantavirus* infection. Early diagnostic studies, however, rule out *Hantavirus*. Subsequently, it is determined that she had a bacterial lung infection with an exacerbation of COPD. She responds to therapy and continues to improve throughout her hospitalization. The student begins care on day 4 of her hospitalization.

Significant Case Concerns: Mrs. Begay is a traditional Navajo living and working on a reservation. She speaks both Navajo and English. Her family and culture are very important and are an integral component of not only planning her care, but in caring for her during this hospitalization.

VCE Workbook Table of Contents

Each lesson has an Ignatavicius & Workman *textbook* reading assignment and activities based on "visiting" the patients in the virtual hospital. The lessons in the workbook provide an opportunity for the student to "practice" what he or she learns from the textbook.

(The chapter[s] in parentheses indicate the reading assignment from the Ignatavicius & Workman *textbook.*)

Getting Started

Getting Set Up
A Quick Tour
A Detailed Tour

Part I – The Virtual Experience: One-Case Lessons

Patient: Carmen Gonzales

Lesson 1 Diabetes Mellitus (Chapter 65)
Lesson 2 Peripheral Arterial Disease (Chapter 36)
Lesson 3 Cultural Aspects of Care (Chapter 6)
Lesson 4 Congestive Heart Failure (Chapter 35)
Lesson 5 Care of Older Adults (Chapter 5)
Lesson 6 Community Care (Chapter 2)
Lesson 7 Evaluation of Care (Chapters 35, 36 & 65)

Patient: Sally Begay

Lesson 8 Pneumonia (Chapters 27 & 31)
Lesson 9 Pain (Chapter 7)
Lesson 10 Cultural Aspects of Care (Chapter 6)
Lesson 11 Chronic Bronchitis and Tuberculosis (Chapters 30 & 31)
Lesson 12 Complementary Therapies (Chapter 4)
Lesson 13 Community Care (Chapter 2)
Lesson 14 Evaluation of Care (Chapters 31 & 32)

Patient: Ira Bradley

Lesson 15 HIV/AIDS (Chapter 22)
Lesson 16 Pain (Chapter 7)
Lesson 17 Cultural Aspects of Care (Chapter 6)
Lesson 18 Malnutrition (Chapter 61)
Lesson 19 End-of-Life Issues (Chapter 9)
Lesson 20 Community Care (Chapter 2)
Lesson 21 Evaluation of Care (Chapter 22)

Patient: David Ruskin

Lesson 22 Fracture (Chapter 52)
Lesson 23 Closed Head Trauma (Chapter 42)
Lesson 24 Cultural Aspects of Care (Chapter 6)
Lesson 25 Pulmonary Embolism and Adult Respiratory Distress Syndrome (Chapter 32)
Lesson 26 Case Management (Chapter 3)
Lesson 27 Community Care (Chapter 2)
Lesson 28 Evaluation of Care (Chapter 52)

Patient: Andrea Wang

Lesson 29 Spinal Cord Injury (Chapter 43)
Lesson 30 Autonomic Dysreflexia and Urinary Retention (Chapter 43)
Lesson 31 Cultural Aspects of Care (Chapter 6)
Lesson 32 Case Management (Chapter 3)
Lesson 33 Rehabilitation (Chapter 10)
Lesson 34 Community Care (Chapter 2)
Lesson 35 Evaluation of Care (Chapter 43)

Part II – The Virtual Experience: Two-Case Lessons

Answer Guidelines for Case Studies

Chapter 17. Case Study for the Preoperative Client

1. Explain to the client that it is possible to have a transfusion of the client's own blood. Because the client's present Hgb and Hct are low, a preoperative blood donation is not possible. The choice for this client would be an intraoperative autologous transfusion and postoperative blood salvage through blood collection during the operative procedure. The advantages of this type of transfusion are guaranteed compatibility and the elimination of the risk of transmission of other bloodborne diseases.
2. The nurse should evaluate the following: the client's understanding of the surgical procedure and postoperative care, the presence of any preexisting diseases or disorders, the current and previous medications, any previous surgeries, the present psychological status, the normalcy of lab work, and others.
3. The client will be taught to do deep exhaling to eliminate inhaled gases. The client should follow the five steps of deep breathing found in Chart 17-6. In regard to vaginal discharge, the client should be taught to expect slight to moderate vaginal bleeding (less than one saturated pad in 4 hours).

Chapter 18. Case Study for the Intraoperative Client

1. Yes, it is possible to develop occipital eschar (pressure breakdown) while positioned in the supine position for as long as open-heart surgery would take. The client does not change position during the procedure, and the head is in direct contact with the mattress. Blood flow may be compromised in the area due to the change in circulation brought about by the need for the heart-lung bypass machine.
2. Notify your nurse manager and educational coordinator so that they can determine whether there is any factual basis to what your friend has said, and, if so, then a corrective plan could be developed and implemented.
3. Pressure breakdown can usually be prevented with a combination of appropriate type and amount of padding, as well as routine shifts of pressure throughout the surgical procedure.

Chapter 19. Case Study for the Postoperative Client

1. Go to the client's room and perform an initial postoperative assessment (see Chart 19-1). By performing a quick head-to-toe assessment of the client, you will be able to gather enough information to determine whether the client is presently at risk for any life-threatening problems. As soon as possible, review the recovery room record.
2. Introduce yourself to the client, stating you are a nurse and you are here to help make his stay go as smoothly as possible. Do not discuss the lack of notice or report or any feelings you have related to this incident with the client.
3. Check the client's medical record to review the postanesthesia care record and check any progress notes or orders. Once you are sure that the client is not in any immediate danger, check with other staff from your unit and with the postanesthesia care unit regarding the breakdown in communication. Develop a plan to improve communication between the units to prevent further breakdown of communication in the future.

Chapter 21. Case Study for the Client with Systemic Lupus Erythematosus

1.
   - Have you been more tired or fatigued lately?
   - Have you had any skin problems other than the facial rash?
   - When did you notice the rash and achy joint?
   - Do other joints hurt?
2. Fever, weakness, fatigue, discoid lesions
3. Childbearing-aged woman who recently had a major stress to her body (such as birth)
4. Antinuclear antibody (ANA) titer, rheumatoid factor, erythrocyte sedimentation rate (ESR)

Chapter 22. Case Study for the Client with AIDS

1. Sample questions that you might ask include:
   - How long have you had chest pain/difficulty breathing?

- Do you have a cough? Do you cough up any sputum? What color is it? What makes the chest pain better? Worse?
- Do the chest pains radiate to any other area?

2. Other physical parameters you want to assess are:
   - Blood pressure
   - Pulse
   - Temperature
   - Skin color
   - Mental status changes
   - Capillary refill

   Rationale: The client is immune compromised and most likely has developed pneumonia.
3. The first thing to do is assist the client to a sitting position to facilitate breathing. Provide a pillow to use as a splint during coughing to reduce chest pain. Contact the primary care provider with a report of your assessment findings, and follow up on telephone orders.

Chapter 28. Case Study for the Client Receiving Oxygen Therapy

1. Because of the critical nature of maintaining airway patency and breathing, assessing Mr. Moss becomes a high priority, especially if the only information you have is that he is having trouble breathing. You should still take the time to maintain sterility of the IV medication. If another nurse is available, you could ask that nurse to go to Mr. Moss's room (tell the nurse what his call was about) while you finish hanging the IV medication, if it is only going to take you another 30 to 60 seconds.
2. Check to see that the nasal cannula is properly placed in the nostrils, the liter flow is turned on at the prescribed flow rate, there are no kinks in the tubing, and oxygen is remaining in the oxygen source (i.e., the tank hasn't run out).

Chapter 29. Case Study for the Client with Vocal Cord Paralysis

1. Assessment information you need to document:
   - Presenting signs and symptoms
   - Respiratory status
   - Client's mental status
   - Data and time of coughing incident
   - Use of accessory muscles
2. Additional assessment data to be collected and documented:
   - Vital signs
   - Auscultation of breath sounds
   - Presence of sputum (color, consistency, content, amount)
   - Using a dental mirror (laryngeal mirror), inspect the client's oral cavity and view the vocal cords. Ask the client to speak while you are observing. Determine whether both cords move to the center during speech.
   - Observe pharynx for redness or swelling.
   - Ask the client and wife when the voice sound changed.
   - Ask the client whether he has any throat soreness.
   - Check the status of the client's advance directives, specifically, is there a DNR (do not resuscitate) request?
3. Priority nursing actions to be implemented include:
   - Reassure the client and wife that coughing episode was a mild choking and not a cold.
   - Notify the primary health care provider of the episode.
   - Tell the client and wife that pressure from the tumor is preventing the vocal cord from closing properly so that the throat is now always open.
   - Teach the client and wife aspiration precautions:
     —Eat and drink only in the upright position.
     —Do not eat or drink when sleepy.
     —Hold breath while swallowing.
     —Avoid small, hard foods such as peanuts, hard candy, raw carrot bites, etc.
     —Have someone stay with the client whenever he eats or drinks.
   - Teach client and family about alternate communication:
     —Have a bell within the client's reach so that he can call for assistance without exertion.
     —Tell the client and wife that the client's voice will not improve, and it will be necessary to keep environmental noise to a minimum when the client speaks to avoid exertion.
     —If feasible, a small battery-powered microphone may be used to increase the client's voice volume for communication.
   - Arrange for the loan of portable suction equipment.
4. Expected outcomes for this situation:
   - The client is expected to verbalize a reduction of anxiety.
   - The client and wife can explain the aspiration precautions.
   - Before you leave the home, the client and family will set up a means for the client to call for assistance.

- The client is expected to maintain a patent airway.

Chapter 30. Case Study for the Client with Chronic Obstructive Pulmonary Disease

1. • When was the onset of symptoms, and what was the duration of symptoms? Do you experience any associated discomfort? Does anything make the symptoms better or worse? Does anyone you are associated with have similar symptoms?
   - Have you ever been told you had a respiratory problem or disease such as asthma, bronchitis, emphysema, cystic fibrosis, or tuberculosis?
   - Have you been exposed to tuberculosis?
   - What type of job do you have?
   - How many pillows do you sleep on?
   - Have you noticed a sudden change in weight or swelling in your ankles?
2. Auscultation of heart and lung sounds, assessment of signs of cyanosis (circumoral, nail bed, mucous membranes), temperature, use of accessory muscles
3. Asthma, occupational asthma, chronic airflow limitation, congestive heart failure, acute viral respiratory infection, tuberculosis, or cancer
4. • Place client in a comfortable semi-Fowler's position, or allow the client to seek the position of most comfort.
   - If the oxygen saturation is less than 90%, the physician may order ABGs and oxygen.
   - The physician will order a bronchodilator for inhalation.
   - Unless there are signs of a bacterial infection, no antibiotics will be prescribed.
5. • Smoking cessation: effects of smoking tobacco, community resources available, and provide encouragement
   - Metered-dose inhaler technique
   - Self-monitoring of peak expiratory flows if asthma is suspected. The client should obtain and record measurements in the early morning and the evening.
   - Provide information regarding the disease process, avoidance of irritants, signs and symptoms of infection, and prevention of infection.
   - Ensure that the client understands when to return for follow-up.

Chapter 30. Case Study for the Client with Lung Cancer

1. Treatment—Stage IIIb patients are not considered surgical candidates. Due to G.F's overall good health, combination therapy with chemotherapy and radiation therapy was suggested as a treatment action. (In this case, chemotherapy with Etoposide 50 mg/m^2 IV over 4 hr/day 1 to 4 times per month, and Cisplatin 100 mg/m^2 IV over 2 hr/day once per month were chosen in combination with radiation of 54 Gy over 3 weeks.)
2. Based on this treatment regimen, the nurse provides client/family education related to diagnosis, chemotherapy agents, and radiation therapy, including self-management and care during therapy. Special attention should be given to the management of potential side effects of chemotherapy, including bone marrow suppression, nausea, constipation, neurotoxicities, alopecia, and anaphylactic reactions. Premedication with antiemetics and hydration should be discussed. The nurse informs the client that his hematologic profile with differential and renal function will be followed up carefully throughout therapy. Potential problems associated with radiation, especially skin care, anorexia, and esophageal mucositis are discussed, and measures to minimize their effects are initiated. The nurse should also include information regarding nutrition, including small frequent meals, complex carbohydrates, and the avoidance of spicy or irritating foods.
3. The nurse recognizes the psychosocial issues that B.F. and his family are facing. Written information is provided to reinforce health teaching relating to the treatment plan. Contact personnel responsible for administering chemotherapy and radiation therapy in the outpatient setting are provided. Information regarding various educational and support programs offered by the American Cancer Society are provided. The National Cancer Institute's Information Service (1-800-4-CANCER) is discussed as an available resource to answer further questions regarding treatment and support services.

Chapter 31. Case Study for the Client with Tuberculosis

1. Ms. Chapel must be placed in Airborne Precautions, preferably in a room designated for TB, or a room known to have the proper 6 circulations of air per minute with ventilation to the outside. If

that type of room is not available, a HEPA filter must be placed in the room (these units can be rented if the hospital does not own one). She is placed in Airborne Precautions because the organism that causes TB is spread via the droplet route.
2. The sputum most likely to contain the highest number of organisms is best collected in the early morning. Saliva will dilute the specimen, but a tiny bit of saliva will not affect the results significantly.
3. Ms. Chapel's children and mother need to be tested for TB infection and, if possible, evaluated for active TB. Prophylactic antibiotic therapy will be initiated if any member of the household is either infected or active. Any other close friends or family members should be counseled regarding the importance of TB testing for them as well. The home should be evaluated for proper ventilation. Ms. Chapel's mother needs to maintain her health and an evaluation of how her health needs are being met should be done. Teach the client, family, and any extended family the importance of good handwashing.

Chapter 32. Case Study for the Client with ARDS

1. His arterial blood gases indicate respiratory and metabolic acidosis as well as refractory hypoxemia. Because he is on 100% oxygen, his Pao_2 should be far greater as calculated by the alveolar air equation (up to 650 mm Hg); instead it is 40 mm Hg.
2. The treatment for refractory hypoxemia is positive and expiratory pressure (PEEP). He should also be sedated to prevent bucking the ventilator, as well as chemically paralyzed to decreased oxygen requirements until his oxygenation status has improved.
3. The higher colloid osmotic pressure in the secretions indicates proteins pulled into the interstitial and alveolar spaces from the capillaries. This is one of the hallmarks of ARDS.

Chapter 35. Case Study for the Client with Heart Failure

1. Limit the questions you ask if your client is having difficulty breathing. Sample questions you might ask include:
   - Do you have chest discomfort?
   - How long have you been feeling ill?
   - What were you doing when this feeling began?
   - Have you felt this way before? If so, when?
   - Do you wake up at night with shortness of breath?
2. Physical assessments you should perform include:
   - Auscultating her lungs, noting respiratory rate, depth, and effort
   - Checking BP
   - Checking pulse oximetry reading (if available)
   - Checking for jugular vein distention and peripheral edema
   - Checking for mental status changes
   - Assessment for presence of ascites

   You should perform these assessments because the client has a history of heart failure and her appearance is suggestive of heart failure and the development of atrial fibrillation.
3. Because the resident's BP is adequate, the first thing you should do is raise the head of the bed to facilitate breathing, followed by oxygen administration. You might initially deliver low-flow O_2 (1 or 2 liters by nasal cannula) because she has a history of COPD and might have a high $Paco_2$. However, don't be surprised if later you are asked to deliver a higher concentration of oxygen to relieve hypoxemia. You need to contact the physician with a report of your findings. Have a staff member stay with the resident to help allay her anxiety and monitor her condition. Be prepared to administer morphine to help allay the client's anxiety.

Chapter 37. Case Study for the Client with Hypovolemic Shock

1. Other assessment techniques you might perform include:
   - Pulse oximetry for oxygen saturation
   - Capillary refill
   - Abdominal assessment (girth, bowel sounds, symmetry, evidence of bruising, palpation for consistency, and subjective signs of tenderness or pain)
   - Any obvious signs of bleeding
2. While hemorrhage could occur anywhere, the most obvious areas to examine include:
   - Perineal area for vaginal bleeding
   - Under the client
   - The IV site

   Hemorrhage is most likely to be internal in this situation. The client's complaint of back pain is consistent with internal hemorrhage. The skin on the lower back may be discolored.
3. Other data to gather might include:
   - Preoperative and operative vital signs

- Any history of bleeding or coagulation disorders
- Types of anesthesia used
- Analgesics administered
- Whether blood was typed and cross-matched
- Mental status changes from baseline
- Any signs of petechiae on the chest

4. Action priorities:
   - Elevate the head of the bed 15 degrees and start oxygen administration by mask.
   - Notify the surgeon/house staff/anesthetist of your findings.
   - Check to see whether the IV line is patent. If it is patent, infuse fluid at 100 mL/hr. If is is not patent, or if venous access is in place, start an IV with 0.9% saline.
   - If blood has not been typed and cross-matched, draw and send a sample for at least two units of blood.
5. Expected outcomes for this situation:
   - The client should have improved oxygenation as evidenced by pink oral mucous membranes and a peripheral oxygen saturation of 95%.
   - The source of the hemorrhage will be identified.
   - The client's vital signs will not worsen before the appropriate surgical intervention is initiated.
   - Appropriate surgical invention will be initiated.

Chapter 42. Case Study for the Client with Central Nervous System Disorders

1. Assessments include a neurologic evaluation, including a mini-mental status exam, a functional assessment to determine his ADL ability, an assessment of the home environment, and an evaluation of the knowledge level of the caregivers. The nurse should also assess the safety of the home environment.
2. Phenytoin is an antiepileptic drug being used to treat the client's seizures. The nurse assesses the family's knowledge regarding the expected effect of the drug, the side effects, and when the health care provider should be called. The client also needs to have frequent monitoring of serum drug levels to ensure therapeutic levels and indications of toxicity. Teaching should also include the fact that the frequency and dosages of the medication should not be changed.
3. The nurse observes the client and documents the seizure activity as described in Charts 42-4 and 42-5 of the textbook.

Chapter 43. Case Study for the Client with a Lumbar Diskectomy

1. A herniated nucleus pulposus (HNP) is sometimes referred to as a "slipped disk." The fall that John experienced caused part of the cartilage between two of his spinal vertebrae to become dislodged. The cartilage was pressing on a spinal nerve and needed to be removed to prevent pain and, perhaps, permanent damage. It will be helpful for the nurse to have or draw a picture to help explain this to the client and his wife.
2. Priorities in care include assessing the surgical site for cerebrospinal leakage or bleeding; performing frequent neurologic checks, including ensuring that John can move and feel his lower extremities and void spontaneously; assessing and managing postoperative pain; body alignment and positioning to prevent stress on the surgical area; and assessment of reflexes.
3. John should keep his back straight and move his trunk as one unit, being careful not to bend at the waist.
4. The only referral will probably be physical therapy on an ambulatory basis. His major limitation will be to avoid lifting and driving for 4 to 6 weeks. He may not return to work until permitted by the surgeon—for at least 6 weeks postoperatively.

Chapter 44. Case Study for the Client with Guillain-Barré Syndrome

1. The nurse should be concerned about possible respiratory compromise if the weakness continues to ascend. Ventilator support may be needed if respiratory muscles are affected.
2. Most often clients have a recent history of an acute illness, especially a respiratory or gastrointestinal infection. Other risk factors include surgery, trauma, or immunization 1 to 8 weeks before the onset of the disease.
3. The nurse should first reassure the client that she will be monitored carefully for progression of the disease. GBS is a peripheral nervous system disease that affects the myelin of the neurons, most often in an ascending pattern. In most cases, the illness is self-limiting and the client can expect a full recovery. In less than 10% of cases, clients experience a chronic or recurrent form of GBS.

Chapter 45. Case Study for the Client with a Head Injury

1. Medications might include Colace, Zantac, Mannitol, Dilantin, Nimodopine, Fentanyl, Codeine, Decadron, and IV fluids.
2. Avoid clustering nursing interventions. Elevate the head of the bed 30 to 45 degrees, maintain normothermia, and avoid neck and extreme hip flexion. Also avoid isometric exercises, noxious stimuli, pain, emotional distress, and muscle exertion. Consider hyperventilation prior to more stressful nursing interventions.
3. Referrals will be needed for physical therapy, occupational therapy, social work, home health, psychological counseling, and a head injury support group. Speech/language therapy may be necessary if speech is impaired. Case management referral will also be needed for continuity of care into the community.
4. When Ann fell from the balcony, one of the arteries in her brain tore and produced a blood clot that put pressure on her brain. The brain began to swell and become inflamed, causing her to become unresponsive. The pressure was relieved by surgery when the clot was removed. Medications were given in the ICU to continue control of the pressure. The brain has no room for swelling without placing additional pressure on the brain's softer tissues.

Chapter 47. Case Study for the Client with Acute Angle-Closure Glaucoma

1. Other assessment techniques you might perform are:
   - Closely inspect the left eye, comparing all features with those of the right eye.
   - Check hand grasps and balance to determine whether other neurologic signs are present.
   - Assess mental status for orientation to time, place, and person.
   - If you are proficient with an ophthalmoscope, check the red reflex, color, and character of the aqueous humor.
2. Questions you should ask might include:
   - What specific activity were you doing when you first became aware of the problem?
   - Has this happened before? If so, when?
   - Are you taking any medications (prescription or over-the-counter)? If so, what?
   - How is your vision now in the left eye compared to the vision in the right eye and your normal left eye vision?
   - Do you see any halos, glare, flashing lights, or dark spots?
3. Plan of action:
   Help her calm down and stop crying. Keep her in a sitting position, do not have her lie down. Ask whether she has an ophthalmologist. If she does, contact the doctor and relate your findings. If she does not, send her to the nearest emergency department (if not in your building, by cab or have someone else drive her). Document the incident, including activities immediately preceding the event, and your findings in the employee record.
4. Expected outcomes:
   - The woman is expected to comply with emergency medical care immediately.
   - The woman is expected to retain her current level of vision.

Chapter 49. Case Study for the Client with External Otitis

1. Additional information necessary for a thorough history includes:
   - Possible changes in hearing
   - Dizziness or tinnitus
   - Hygiene practices, such as bathing, changes in hair care products, ear cleaning techniques
   - Participation in sports, particularly swimming
   - History of external otitis and possible past etiologies
2. Physical signs of external otitis include:
   - Pain with manipulation of left pinna
   - Ear canal edematous, erythematous, and possibly occluded
   - Drainage from affected ear canal
   - Intact tympanic membrane with normal landmarks, if able to visualize
   - No tenderness over mastoid process or enlargement of local lymph nodes
   - No constitutional signs or symptoms: fever, malaise, anorexia
3. Teaching or reinforce prevention of external otitis include:
   - Proper administration of topical antibiotics to treat external otitis.
   - Proper canal drying techniques after water sports or bathing
   - Proper canal hygiene to remove excessive cerumen
   - Avoiding placing any objects in ear canal

4. Expected outcomes specific to this situation include:
   - Decrease in pain within 24 hours
   - Decrease in ear drainage within 48 hours
   - Compliance with medication regimen
   - Client will be able to demonstrate proper canal hygiene on unaffected ear

Chapter 51. Case Study for the Client with Acute Osteomyelitis

1. - Assess the nature of the wound, including location, size, and presence of drainage or ulceration.
   - Assess the neurovascular status of the foot.
   - Assess the client's knowledge level regarding foot care for diabetics.
2. - Leukocyte count
   - Erythrocyte sedimentation rate
   - Wound culture and sensitivity
   - Blood glucose
   - Bone scan
3. Frequent dressing changes, antibiotic therapy, and health teaching about diabetes, wound care, and drug therapy

Chapter 52. Case Study for the Client with a Fractured Hip

1. Do a head-to-toe assessment to make sure that she has no life-threatening problems, such as a head injury. Check her vital signs and try to determine why and how she fell. Check her legs for equal length. Shortening of the affected leg is common when a hip fracture occurs.
2. Tell her that you will be sure that someone goes with her to the hospital. Also reassure her that everyone is different, and that her friend may have had other medical problems that contributed to her death.
3. She will probably have an open reduction with internal fixation surgery, then return to the nursing home for rehabilitation.

Chapter 54. Case Study for the Client with Oral Cavity Cancer

1. Overuse of tobacco and alcohol is the primary cause of carcinomas. The nurse should assess the client's tobacco use in all forms and his history of alcohol consumption. Methods of eliminating these habits from the client's lifestyle should be discussed.
2. The nurse should assess the client's level of fear and anxiety about cancer. Some clients fear death; others fear pain and loss of family roles. The meaning of cancer to the client is also important.
3. The nurse instructs the client undergoing composite resection about:
   - The probability of having a tracheostomy and the required nursing care for a tracheostomy (oxygen therapy and sectioning)
   - The temporary loss of speech because of the tracheostomy
   - The need for vital signs to be taken frequently postoperatively
   - The need to take nothing by mouth for 7 to 10 days
   - The need to have intravenous (IV) lines in place for 2 to 3 days
   - Postoperative medications and activity (out of bed on the first postoperative day)
   - Any drains involved (surgical drains, Foley catheter)

Chapter 55. Case Study for the Client with Gastroesophageal Reflux Disease (GERD)

1. Sample questions you should ask include:
   - Are your symptoms worse at night?
   - What are your specific symptoms?
   - How long have you had symptoms?
   - Are you taking any medications other than Motrin?
   - What do you do to relieve the pain?
   - Do you smoke?
   - Do you drink beverages that contain caffeine?
2. Instructions you might want to mention in a teaching plan for the client with GERD include:
   - Stop smoking because nicotine decreases LES tone.
   - Avoid drinking caffeinated coffee, tea, and cola beverages.
   - Don't wear restrictive clothing.
   - Lose weight (if obese) to improve symptoms.
   - Sleep with the head of the bed elevated.
   - Eat small meals.
   - Don't eat within 3 hours of going to bed.
   - Avoid heavy lifting or working in a bent-over position.

Chapter 56. Case Study for the Client with Peptic Ulcer Disease (PUD)

1. Sample questions might include:
   - How and what have you been eating and drinking in the past few weeks?
   - How long have you been experiencing these symptoms?
   - How much alcohol do you consume?
   - How much and how often do you take ibuprofen?
   - Have you ever experienced symptoms like this in the past? If so, how did you manage the symptoms?
   - How often and how much antacid do you take?
   - Have you noticed any change in the character of your stool, except for the color change?

   You might also encourage her to discuss past and ongoing stressors, but don't assume the computer conversion has been a stressor.
2. Components of physical assessment include:
   - Vital signs, including postural blood pressure check
   - Abdominal assessment
   - Stool for occult blood

   It is important to rule out active GI bleeding. A significant drop in blood pressure amy indicate blood loss.
3. Her stools should be assessed for occult blood. She should also have a hemoglobin and hematocrit assessment because she could have active GI bleeding.

Chapter 57. Case Study for the Client with a Bowel Obstruction

1. Sample questions might include:
   - When did your bowels last move?
   - When and how muck milk of magnesia did you take last?
   - Have you experienced any nausea or vomiting?
   - How has your appetite been?
   - Have you experienced any abdominal pain?
2. The components of the physical examination should include:
   - An abdominal assessment
   - Vital signs
   - A respiratory assessment
3. Problems the client may be experiencing include severe constipation or a bowel obstruction.
4. His immobility, chronic constipation history, and history of abdominal surgery place him at risk for a bowel obstruction.
5. The most appropriate nursing action is to refer the client to his health care provider immediately.

Chapter 58. Case Study for the Client with Inflammatory Bowel Disease

1. The priority is her physical complaints. Although her anxiety may be contributing to her symptoms, her physiologic integrity is a higher priority.
2. You would ask her how much she has had to drink, whether she feels nauseated or has vomited, whether she is passing gas through her stoma, and when these symptoms first started.
3. You would want to perform a complete abdominal assessment including auscultating bowel sounds, assessing the stoma and its effluence, and inspecting and palpating the abdomen. You would also want to assess her vital signs and respiratory function.
4. You should first attend to her physical needs. Encourage her to stay in bed, and offer her an emesis basin. Next, you should contact the surgeon regarding your assessment findings.

Chapter 59. Case Study for the Client with Cirrhosis

1. He is probably experiencing hepatic encephalopathy caused by a buildup of ammonia.
2. Assessment data include a complete neurologic assessment, with a focus on level of consciousness and mental status. A serum ammonia level is the essential laboratory data.
3. Medications used include lactulose and neomycin. Both of these medications reduce the nitrogenous waste load within the intestines, and thereby lower the ammonia level.

Chapter 60. Case Study for the Client with Acute Pancreatitis

1. You are monitoring for changes indicative of hypovolemia, a common complication associated with acute pancreatitis.
2. The client may find that the fetal position helps to decrease pain.
3. Meperidine hydrochloride (Demerol) is the drug of choice because it supposedly causes less inci-

dence of spasm of the pancreatic ducts and sphincter of Oddi than other opioids such as morphine.
4. She may be experiencing a paralytic ileus.

Chapter 63. Case Study for the Client with Acromegaly and Hypophysectomy

1. Explain that hypophysectomy will reduce his hormone levels and may improve his sexual functioning. His hepatomegaly and the growth in his head, hands, and feet may not improve. You should explain to him that he will have nasal packing for 2 to 3 days and that this will necessitate mouth breathing. You must emphasize that he cannot cough, sneeze, bend over at the waist, or brush his teeth after surgery. He will receive medication for pain. Ice packs may be used in the early hours following surgery.
2. Postoperatively, you will want to monitor the following:
   - Neurologic status
   - Fluid balance (intake and output)
   - Pulmonary status (encourage deep breathing but not coughing)
   - Nasal drainage for CSF by testing drainage for glucose
   - Bowel movement to prevent constipation and thus avoid straining
   - Blood loss
3. Complications you should be alert to are the development of diabetes insipidus and CSF leak. Infection also is a possibility.
4. Home care teaching should include:
   - Avoid bending at the waist.
   - Avoid straining to have a bowel movement. Suggest a high-fiber diet and stool softeners.
   - Avoid tooth brushing for 1 to 2 weeks and encourage use of mouthwash or dental floss.
   - Instructions about hormone replacement—vasopressin, cortisol, thyroid, and gonadal hormones.
5. The following outcomes can be expected for this situation:
   - Intracranial pressure will remain without normal limits.
   - The client will remain infection-free.
   - Bowel movements will be soft, occur daily, and be passed easily.
   - The client will comply with the prescribed medication regimen and postoperative activity restrictions.
   - Within 8 weeks after surgery, the client will be able to resume a level of sexual functioning equivalent to that experienced before the onset of hyperpituitarism.
   - The client will experience an improvement in body image.

Chapter 64. Case Study for the Client with Graves' Disease

1. You would check her serum calcium and electrolytes immediately. Tingling around the mouth is a sign of hypocalcemia and leads to tetany, a life-threatening emergency.
2. Other physical assessment data include:
   - Checking for hemorrhage behind the neck
   - Asking the client to speak every 1 to 2 hours to assess for laryngeal nerve damage or tracheal edema
   - Checking for muscle weakness and tingling in toes. You need this additional data to check for bleeding that may not be apparent on the front of the neck. Gravity makes the blood flow back behind the neck. Hoarseness that worsens after surgery is an indication of laryngeal nerve damage, and asking the client to speak every 2 hours can determine a change in the voice. Muscle weakness and tingling can be a sign of hypocalcemia, a serious complication of thyroid surgery.
3. You ensure a tracheostomy tray and a pair of clip removers are at the bedside after surgery, should there be a large amount of edema causing airway impairment.
4. The following expected outcomes are desired in this situation:
   - No postoperative hemorrhage
   - Client able to maintain a normal breathing pattern
   - Serum calcium levels remain normal
   - Deep tendon reflexes are normal
   - Trousseau's and Chvostek's signs are negative

Chapter 65. Cast Study for the Client with Diabetes and Visual Impairment

1. Precautions for prevention of hypoglycemia include:
   - Maintain adequate dietary intake.
   - Exercise extreme care in insulin measurement and administration.
   - Carry a source of glucose with you at all times.
   - Monitor blood glucose with adaptive devices when hypoglycemic symptoms appear; consult

health care provider for values consistently below acceptable ranges.

Precautions for prevention of hyperglycemia include:

- Always take insulin as prescribed.
- Monitor blood glucose with adaptive devices on a regular basis, consult health care provider for values above acceptable ranges.
- Consult medical care provider for signs and symptoms of illness.

2. Ways to alter the environment to aid in measurement of accurate insulin doses include:
   - The nurse recommends that the client improve vision by supplementing overhead fluorescent lighting with an incandescent lamp directed toward the work space.
   - Placing the clear insulin syringe against a dark background provides color contrast that will enhance vision.
   - Some means of separating the NPH insulin from the regular insulin bottle is necessary so that errors in measurement are not made. Coding the vials of insulin with bright colors or using felt-tipped markers will aid in identification of the correct bottle to be used.
   - Bringing the insulin syringe close to the eye makes it easier to see.
   - Even though the client has been taking insulin injections for some time, the nurse may provide written materials to stress some points on injection technique. Material that is printed with an enlarged typeface is easier to read.
3. Critical points that would be involved in a teaching session on adaptive devices for use with insulin syringes include:
   - Different types of insulin need to be identified by an added tactile label. The label needs to be attached in such a way that the type of insulin and expiration date are easily identified.
   - Proper placement of the device on the syringe is essential for correct measurements.
   - The insulin bottle needs to be held upright when measuring insulin.
   - Air can be expelled from the syringe by pulling a small amount of insulin into the syringe, moving the plunger in and out three times, and measuring insulin on the fourth draw.
   - A system to determine how many doses can be drawn from a bottle of insulin needs to be established so that the client with visual impairment does not inject air from an empty bottle rather than insulin.

Chapter 67. Case Study for the Client with a *Candida* Skin Infection

1. Methods of obtaining assessment information that you need to collect include:
   - Inspect other skin-fold areas (under arms and breasts) for rash.
   - Obtain a history of the present problem from the daughter:
     - —How long has the client been incontinent of urine?
     - —Is the client also incontinent of feces?
     - —When did she (the daughter) first observe a problem with the skin?
     - —Has she been treating it with anything?
   - Formulate a detailed description of the rash including, in addition to the information in the case study, the size and shape of the various lesions.
2. Additional skin assessment data that need to be collected and documented include:
   - Condition of the skin over all bony prominences, with particular attention to sacrum, ischial tuberosities, and trochanteric prominences (where moisture combined with immobility may accelerate ulcer formation)
   - Braden risk assessment score
   - General skin integrity (collect data regarding skin tears, excessive dryness on lower legs, abnormal lesions, and other skin problems associated with aging)
3. Priority nursing actions that need to be implemented include:
   - Client/family teaching, instructing the daughter to:
     - —Remove briefs and leave skin open to air when client is in bed (briefs hold moisture against skin); use underpads to protect linen.
     - —Clean skin gently with mild soap and water after each episode of incontinence; pat dry.
     - —Use zinc oxide–based ointment as a moisture barrier cream, apply to all areas of involvement after cleansing, and use mineral oil or vegetable oil to remove cream when cleansing (requires less friction).
     - —Reposition frequently (every 2 hours while awake) for maximum circulation to perineal area.
     - —Inspect bony prominences and take measures, such as positioning and padding, to relieve/reduce pressure.

Notify primary care provider of your findings and obtain orders for:
- Urine culture (to rule out UTI as a contributing factor for incontinence)
- Topical antifungal cream (to be applied PRN under moisture barrier cream)
- Overbed cradle (to tent sheets and promote air circulation while providing privacy)
- Pressure relief mattress if the client has a moderate to high risk for pressure-related skin problems (Braden risk score)
- Nursing aide to come to home daily (to assist with personal hygiene and help daughter to get client out of bed in chair)

4. Expected outcomes for this situation:
   - The daughter is expected to comply with skin care regimen.
   - The daughter is expected to demonstrate skill in assessing skin condition, using appropriate skin-cleansing techniques, and applying recommended topical agents.
   - The mother's rash is expected to resolve within 1 week of initiating the skin care regimen.
   - Each open area on the mother's perineum is expected to decrease in size or close within 1 week.

Chapter 68. Case Study for the Client with a Burn Injury

1. Initial physical assessment techniques include:
   - Inspection, which indicates:
     —Burns of the face, head, neck, and carbon particles around the nose, indicators of high risk for direct airway injury
     —Circumferential burns of both arms and both legs, which are indicators of high risk for altered tissue perfusion, peripheral
     —Shortness of breath and "incoherent" speech, which may indicate altered brain tissue perfusion
   - Auscultation to determine the quality of breath sounds and bowel sounds listening especially for wheezing or stridor
   - Palpation to establish the quality of circulation distal to the circumferential burns of the extremities and to establish baseline vital signs
   - A generalized estimation of the extent of injury using the rule of nines

   Initial interventions should include:
   - Oxygen per nasal cannula
   - Preparation for endotracheal intubation
   - Insertion of an indwelling urinary catheter to accurately measure urine output
   - Establishment of patent intravenous sites for intravenous fluid therapy
   - Beginning of initial integumentary assessment to determine the size and depth of burns
2. Ongoing assessments include:
   - Assessment of cardiac output including urine output, mental status, pulses, blood pressure, and heart rate
   - Assessment of respiratory status to assure adequate breathing patterns and oxygenation
   - Assessment of pain
   - Assessment of peripheral tissue perfusion
   - Assessment of renal function to assure adequate clearance of toxic waste products and to measure the adequacy of fluid resuscitation
   - Assessment of respiratory status, the auscultation of lung sounds
3. Actual and potential problems with interventions that may be done in the acute phase of burn injury are:
   - Risk for Infection—drug therapy, isolation therapy, environmental manipulation, and surgical excision
   - Impaired Skin Integrity—mechanical debridement, enzymatic debridement, burn wound dressing, surgical debridement, and grafting
   - Altered Nutrition—diet therapy, fluid replacement
   - Impaired Mobility—positioning, range-of-motion exercises, ambulation, pressure dressings, and surgical measures to release constricting scar tissue
   - Body Image Disturbance—grief process, decision-making and independent activities, and surgical reconstruction and cosmetic surgery
4. Teaching parameters that should be implemented for the patient and family in the rehabilitation phase include:
   - Dressing changes
   - Signs and symptoms of infection
   - Medication regimens
   - Use of prosthetic and positioning devices
   - Correct application and care of pressure garments
   - Comfort measures to reduce pruritus

Chapter 70. Case Study for the Client with Urinary Incontinence

1. The client knows that fluids make urine. She also knows that she has difficulty maintaining conti-

nence, so she limits her fluid intake to limit the amount of urine she makes. She thinks that she will then have less incontinence. She may also be concerned about whether someone will be able to respond to her call in time enough to help get her to the toileting facilities.

2. It is very important for the client to force fluids for several reasons: (1) She has an active infection, pneumonia, even though she is being treated. (2) She is at risk for renal insufficiency. Being elderly, she has reduced renal function as result of the aging process. She is on antibiotics, which in the presence of reduced renal volumes, causes nephrotoxicity. (3) Fluids are important to decrease the viscosity of secretions.
3. You should discuss her concerns over not being able to get to the bathroom quickly enough. Some interventions you could try include getting a bedside commode, having a fracture pan right next to her in the bed, offering toileting opportunities every 1 or 2 hours (depending on how frequently she voids), and reviewing her food and fluid selections to see whether she is selecting any that are known bladder irritants.

Chapter 71. Case Study for the Client with Diabetic Nephropathy

1. Empathize with her. State back to her what she might be feeling, i.e., "You must feel as though you have no control," or "You must feel that all your efforts at trying to control your blood sugars hasn't worked," or "What does it mean to you that you have the disease in your kidneys?"
2. Ask what is it about dialysis that concerns her the most, or ask what she has heard about dialysis. Restate back to her what concerns she seems to be expressing. Assess her understanding of dialysis.
3. The National Kidney Foundation, American Diabetes Association, American Kidney Fund, local support groups, professional counselors

Chapter 72. Case Study for the Client with Acute Renal Failure

1. Risk factors for ARF for this client include: age, hypertension, use of captopril and ibuprofen, possible infection, and possible volume depletion from decreased water ingestion.
2. Measures to prevent ARF for this client include:
   - Close monitoring of laboratory values such as BUN, creatinine, urine specific gravity, and fluid and electrolytes to detect early evidence of ARF
   - Careful assessment of fluid status using intake and output and body weight
   - Prompt correction of volume depletion
   - Careful use of NSAIDs and other known nephrotoxic drugs, especially given this client's age
3. Circumstances that might cause the BUN/creatinine ratio to be elevated in this client are autoregulatory responses (renal vasoconstriction, renin-angiotensin-aldosterone, and release of anti-diuretic hormone) in response to volume depletion and instititial inflammatory changes from infection and nephrotoxic drugs.

Chapter 74. Case Study for the Client Having Breast Surgery

1. Preoperative teaching should focus on preparing the client for the surgical procedure, postoperative management, and their needs. The nurse should assess the client's level of knowledge of the surgical procedure and what the client expects will occur in the postoperative phase. General information related to the operating room and postanesthesia care unit should be reviewed. A teaching plan care should be developed to correct any misconceptions and knowledge deficits. The woman will need information about how advanced the disease is, the likelihood of cure, treatment options and side effects, how it will affect her life and self-image, how family will be affected, and home self-care. The nurse asks the client whether she has known anyone with breast cancer and what type of experience she has had with breast cancer and cancer in general. The nurse should assess for any problems related to sexuality. Care of the woman facing surgery for breast cancer focuses on psychological preparation and preoperative teaching. The issues related to anxiety and lack of knowledge are primary. Significant others should also be included in any discussions. The client should be knowledgeable about the type of procedure. Information to discuss with the patient may include the presence of a drainage device, location of the incision, and mobility restrictions, length of hospital stay, and basic preoperative and postoperative needs of any surgical client. The nurse should supplement any teaching with written instructions.

   Postoperative informational needs of the patient relate to hand and arm care, care of drainage tubes, wound care, and measures available for comfort. When axillary lymph nodes have been removed, procedures such as blood pressure measurements, injections, and venipunctures should be avoided in the affected arm. The client should also be taught other measures to promote lymphatic fluid return such as elevating the arm and beginning exercises and exercise progression. The nurse teaches the client how to empty, measure, and record the drainage from the drainage tubes. The client is taught how to manage the wound and the signs and symptoms of a wound infection. Plans for breast reconstruction and temporary prosthesis should be discussed with the client.

2. The nurse should allow the client to verbalize any feelings about the disease and her choice of treatment. The nurse should provide information related to the various options, including both nonsurgical and surgical options.
3. The need for additional resources should be evaluated for each individual. Referral may be needed for psychological counseling services. Financial concerns may be discussed with social services. Support groups in the community may be helpful for some individuals. A referral can be made to the American Cancer Society's Reach Recovery in either the preoperative or postoperative phase. Health care providers may know other clients with breast cancer who are willing to make a preoperative visit. Additionally, formal and informal community support groups, such as encouragement, normalcy counseling, opportunity, Reaching Out, Energies Revived (ENCORE), may be available.
4. The home care needs of this client relate to health teaching and include: measures to optimize active body image information to enhance interpersonal relationships; exercise to regain full range of motion; measures to prevent infection of the incision; measures to avoid injury, infection, and subsequent swelling of the affected arm; and care of the drainage device.
5. A basic overview of breast cancer should be included in the presentation. This could include information on the major types of breast cancer, etiology, incidence, and risk factors. Emphasis should be on the importance of health maintenance practices. A detailed description of breast self-examination and the role of mammography for screening for breast cancer should be the major focus of the presentation.

Chapter 75. Case Study for the Client Having an Abdominal Hysterectomy

1. A general postoperative assessment should be performed that is similar to that of any client having abdominal surgery. The nurse should assess vital signs, bowel sounds (it is expected that bowel sounds will be present in the immediate postoperative period with a gradual return to normal), and lung sounds. The nurse assesses for vaginal bleeding (there should be less than one saturated pad in 4 hours). The incision site is also assessed for bleeding (a small amount is normal). The incision should be intact and without signs of infection. Urinary output should be assessed and measured (there should be at least 30 mL/hr). A pain assessment should be performed. The nurse observes the patient for any signs of complications associated with TAH.
2.
   - Risk for Fluid Volume Deficit related to trauma from the surgical procedure
   - Risk for Alteration in Urinary Elimination related to surgical trauma
   - Risk for Infection related to the abdominal incision and nonsterile vaginal canal
   - Acute Pain related to the abdominal incision
   - Alteration in Bowel Elimination related to manipulation of the bowel during the surgical procedure
   - Risk for Ineffective Airway Clearance related to shallow breathing patterns secondary to pain
   - Risk for Alteration in tissue perfusion related to immobility and pooling of blood in the pelvic vessels
3. The client should be told to avoid or limit stair climbing for 1 month. To avoid infection and trauma the nurse advises the client to avoid tub baths, tampons, and sexual intercourse for 4 to 6 weeks. Prolonged sitting is avoided to prevent pooling of blood in the pelvic vessels. Strenuous activity, active sports, and heavy lifting are avoided. Driving a car is avoided for 4 to 6 weeks. Physical changes associated with TAH-BSO should be taught. These include cessation of menses, inability to become pregnant, weakness and fatigue, and the symptoms of surgically induced menopause with ovary removal. Foods that promote tissue healing and synthesis of RBCs should be consumed, such as protein, iron, and vitamin C. Signs and symptoms of infection are reviewed with the client. Possible emotional reactions are discussed with the client. If the client is

prescribed hormone replacement therapy, the nurse teaches the client the purpose of this medication and the potential side effects. The client is advised of when follow up care is to be scheduled.

Chapter 77. Case Study for the Client with a Sexually Transmitted Disease

1. Other critical client history information that should be gathered includes:
   - Further information about the current episode including symptom history and self-treatment measures, state of general health, usual health maintenance practices, medical history including major health problems, menstrual problems, and contraceptive history, and sexual history, including type and frequency of activity, number of sexual contacts, and sexual preferences
2. Other physical and laboratory data that should be obtained include vital signs, abdominal examination, and examination of genital, rectal, oral, and pelvic areas, urinalysis, hematology, and samples for microbiology and virology.
3. Assessments/interventions that should be carried out first are: careful explanations for all procedures, reassurance and support during physical examination, nonjudgemental attitude, the physical examination, and any ordered laboratory tests.
4. Assessments/interventions that should be completed in 24 to 48 hours include: pain management with analgesics, sitz baths, heat to lower abdomen, antibiotic therapy, completion of the client history, and the teaching plan.